Information Skills for Nursing Students

Kay Hutchfield

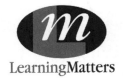

LearningMatters

First published in 2010 by Learning Matters Ltd

© 2010 Kay Hutchfield and Mooi Standing

British Library Cataloguing in Publication Data
A CIP record for this book is available from the British Library

ISBN: 978 1 84445 381 8

This book is also available in the following ebook formats:

Adobe ebook: 978 1 84445 747 2
EPUB ebook: 978 1 84445 746 5
Kindle: 978 0 85725 014 8

The right of Kay Hutchfield and Mooi Standing to be identified as the authors of this Work has been asserted by them in accordance with the Copyright, Designs and Patents Act, 1988.

Cover design by Toucan Design
Project management by Diana Chambers
Typeset by Kelly Winter
Printed and bound in Great Britain by TJ International Ltd, Padstow, Cornwall

Learning Matters Ltd
33 Southernhay East
Exeter EX1 1NX
Tel: 01392 215560
E-mail: info@learningmatters.co.uk
www.learningmatters.co.uk

Contents

Foreword

This excellent book demystifies information skills, giving readers a clear understanding of its relevance in learning to be a nurse and practising nursing, and knowledge of how to develop their skills in both respects. It is an important addition to the *Transforming Nursing Practice* series as accessing, reviewing and applying information underpins the NMC Standards for Pre-registration Nursing Education in relation to both lifelong learning and evidence-based practice. Kay Hutchfield combines her knowledge, understanding and boundless enthusiasm for the subject with her experience as a nurse teacher to skilfully create an accessible, informative, stimulating, rewarding and essential practical guide. The book is written in a straightforward and engaging style which encourages without patronising and stimulates without overloading. Readers will feel that Kay is an ally working alongside them as they progress through the book.

After reading this book nursing students will be able to:

- devise and implement personal development plans to improve their information skills;
- search for information to broaden and deepen their understanding of relevant theory or research;
- identify various types and sources of evidence, where to access and how to evaluate them;
- organise and communicate findings to inform academic work and evidence-based practice;
- bookmark and revisit information-rich websites to continually update their knowledge and skills;
- understand how health informatics innovations enhance efficiency and quality in healthcare.

A key feature of the book are the numerous and varied activities that challenge and enable readers to practise the skills discussed, identify achievable targets so they can honestly self-assess the development of their information skills, and become more competent and confident. This is very helpful in the development and application of transferable graduate skills. *Information Skills for Nursing Students* will greatly benefit beginning students new to higher education and those more experienced, who also need the tools to focus, select and harness relevant information from the infinite array available. I have enjoyed, and learnt a lot from, reading and editing the book, and I highly recommend it.

Mooi Standing
Series Editor

About the author

Kay Hutchfield is a Senior Lecturer in the Department of Health, Wellbeing and the Family at Canterbury Christ Church University, and part of the child nursing teaching team. Between 2004 and 2009 she led an interprofessional module aimed at developing the academic literacy skills of pre-registration students across eight health and social care professions. This role provided insight into some of the specific challenges faced by educators in engaging students in developing their information literary skills and enhancing their ability to access reliable evidence that they can use to inform their assignments and underpin their practice.

Acknowledgements

My thanks go to Faculty Librarians Kate Davies, Karen Worden and Emily Hurt for their help and support in developing my own library skills and teaching material, and to Kate for her valuable feedback on Chapters 2 and 3.

I would also like to thank Su Westerman for involving me in the DEBUT project and her valuable feedback on Chapters 5 and 6.

The author and publisher would like to thank the following for permission to reproduce copyright material:

Table 3.2: Sources of information to support professional practice, pages 43–4. Adapted from Wojciechowicz, L (2010), *Internet for Nursing*, free online tutorial, The Virtual Training Suite (formerly owned by The Intute Consortium). Accessed 31 May 2010 online at **www.vts.intute.ac.uk/tutorial/nursing**.

Screenshots from Microsoft Internet Explorer®, pages 77–8, used with permission from Microsoft. Microsoft and Internet Explorer are either registered trademarks or trademarks of Microsoft Corporation in the United States and/or other countries.

Screenshots from NHS Evidence, pages 77–8, used with permission from NHS Evidence.

Screenshots from Netvibes™, Figures 5.2, 5.3, 5.4 and 5.5, pages 79–81, used with permission from Netvibes.

eBay for use of their logo in a screenshot taken from Netvibes, Figure 5.4, page 81. The eBay logo is a trademark of eBay Inc.

RSS icon, page 82. Usage complies with the Mozilla Foundation RSS feed icon suggested guidelines at **www.mozilla.org/foundation/feed-icon-guidelines**.

Screenshots from Google Reader TM feed reader, Figure 5.6, page 83. Usage covered by Google Inc. permissions policy **www.google.com/permissions**. Google Reader™ feed reader is a trademark of Google Inc.

Every effort has been made to trace all copyright holders within the book, but if any have been inadvertently overlooked, the publisher will be pleased to make the necessary arrangements at the first opportunity.

Introduction

This book introduces you, the nursing student to some of the key transferable graduate skills you will need in order to support your academic studies and your professional development. It aims to provide a practical guide that promotes information literacy skills, and the knowledge and understanding required to develop good study habits that will continue to support your development once you make the transition to being a qualified nurse.

The book also provides an introduction to technology that can make accessing information easier and more efficient. Health informatics is explored and examples are given of IT systems being used to provide patients/clients with a more effective service.

Chapter 1 provides an introduction to key skills, their relevance to studying at university and to professional practice and the place of information skills in this. This includes some discussion of communication and academic writing. It uses a series of self-analysis tools to encourage students to identify areas that may enhance or inhibit their ability to develop successfully academically and professionally. Part of this process includes guidance on the creation of a personal development plan (PDP), which will facilitate the enhancement of the skills necessary to study successfully at university.

Chapter 2 provides an introduction to simple searches for information and offers approaches that can be used to refine or expand such searches. It explores some of the advantages and limitations of searching on the internet, and provides some guidance on keeping records of the search process.

Following on from Chapter 2, Chapter 3 considers some of the types and sources of information nursing students will be expected to access in their search for evidence, in order to support their academic work and underpin their practice. It will consider how these sources can be evaluated, so that the student can have confidence in the credibility of the information accessed.

Chapter 4 focuses on using information effectively in academic work and stresses the importance of developing good reading habits and note-taking skills. Academic writing and paraphrasing are explored alongside consideration of referencing and confidentiality in academic work. The development of a learning contract for practice placements is also considered in order to maximise the learning opportunities available in practice.

Chapter 5 explores systems that are available to enhance the effective storage and retrieval of electronic information. This includes simple methods such as bookmarks to store favourite websites, and personal portals such as Netvibes. The emphasis here is on developing resources for the student that can be easily accessed and can provide sources of reliable information.

Chapter 6 introduces the concept of health informatics and how IT systems are developing to support care delivery, by providing a more efficient way of managing patient information and some routine tasks. It provides insight into NHS Connecting for Health and highlights the need for all nurses to have sufficient IT skills to support the technological advances of the future.

NMC *Standards for Pre-registration Nursing Education*, Essential Skills Clusters and QAA subject benchmark statements

The Nursing and Midwifery Council (NMC) has standards of competence that have to be met by applicants to different parts of the nursing and midwifery register. These standards are what they deem to be necessary for the delivery of safe, effective nursing and midwifery practice.

As well as specific competencies, the NMC identifies specific skills that nursing students must have at various points in their training programme. These Essential Skills Clusters (ESCs) are essential abilities that students need to attain in order to practise to their full potential.

This book identifies some of the competencies and skills within the realm of information skills that student nurses need in order to be entered on to the NMC register. These competencies and ESCs are presented at the start of each chapter so that it is clear which of them the chapter addresses. All of the competencies and ESCs in this book relate to the *generic standards* that all nursing students must achieve. This book includes the latest draft standards for 2010 onwards, taken from the *Standards for Pre-registration Nursing Education: Draft for consultation* (NMC, 2010). For links to the pre-2010 standards, please visit the website for this book at **www.learning matters.co.uk/nursing**. This website will also list any amendments to the standards when the final version is published in autumn 2010.

In addition, some of the chapters are linked to Quality Assurance Agency benchmark statements (QAA, 2008), which are provided for BSc programmes for a range of subjects, including nursing. Subject benchmark statements provide a description of the content of programmes and the general expectations in terms of standards for the award, which include the 'attributes and capabilities' that those achieving the qualification should demonstrate. In addition to the statements themselves (QAA, 2008), the QAA *Health Studies* document (available at **www.qaa.ac.uk/academicinfrastructure/benchmark/ statements/Healthstudieso8.pdf**) contains a reference to transferable skills on page 4.

Activities and tests

At various stages within each chapter there are points at which you can break to undertake activities, which form an important element of your understanding of the content of each chapter. As this is a book on information skills, many of the activities are practical and those in Chapter 5 particularly require you to be logged on to the internet. Where appropriate, there are suggested or potential answers to activities at the end of the chapter. It is recommended that, where possible, you try to engage with the activities in order to increase your understanding of information technology.

In addition to the activities, there is a short test at the end of each chapter to check what you have learnt. This will enable you to ensure that you have understood the content of each chapter, before moving on to the next. Answers are provided at the end of each test.

Chapter 1

Getting ready to study

Draft NMC Standards for Pre-registration Nursing Education

This chapter will address the following draft competencies:

Domain: Professional values

8. All nurses must be responsible and accountable for keeping their own knowledge and skills up-to-date through continuing professional development and life-long learning. They must use evaluation, supervision and appraisal to improve their performance and enhance the safety and quality of care and service delivery.
9. All nurses must recognise the limits of their own competence and knowledge. They must reflect on their own practice and seek advice from, or refer to, other professionals where necessary.

Domain: Communication and interpersonal skills

2. All nurses must use a range of communication skills and technologies to support person-centred care and enhance the quality and safety of healthcare. They must make sure that people receive all the information they need about their care in a language and manner that is right for them, and that allows them to make informed choices and consent to treatment.
3. All nurses must use verbal, non-verbal and written communication to listen, recognise, interpret and record people's knowledge and understanding of their needs. They must share information with others while respecting individual rights to confidentiality.
9. All nurses must maintain accurate, clear and complete written or electronic records using the right kind of language, avoiding jargon, and using plain English so that everyone involved in the care process understands the meaning.

Draft Essential Skills Clusters

This chapter will address the following draft ESCs:

Cluster: Care, compassion and communication

6. People can trust the newly registered nurse to engage therapeutically and actively listen to their needs and concerns, responding using skills that are helpful, providing information that is clear, accurate, meaningful and free from jargon.

Draft Essential Skills Clusters continued

By the first progression point:

i. Communicates effectively both orally and in writing, so that the meaning is always clear.

By entry to the register:

ix. Provides accurate and comprehensive written and verbal reports based on best available evidence.

Cluster: Organisational aspects of care

14. People can trust the newly registered graduate nurse to be autonomous and confident as a member of the multi-displinary or multi-agency team and to inspire confidence in others.

By the second progression point:

v. Communicates with colleagues verbally, face-to-face and by telephone, and in writing and electronically in a way that the meaning is clear, and checks that the communication has been fully understood.

15. People can trust the newly registered graduate nurse to safely delegate to others and to respond appropriately when a task is delegated to them.

By entry to the register:

v. Recognises and addresses deficits in knowledge and skill in self and others and takes appropriate action.

Chapter aims

After reading this chapter, you will be able to:

- understand the nature of key skills and their relevance to studying at university and to professional practice;
- use a series of self-analysis tools to identify areas that may enhance or inhibit your ability to develop successfully your information literacy skills;
- create a personal development plan (PDP) that will facilitate the development and enhancement of the skills necessary to study successfully at university.

Introduction

In 1997, Sir Ron Dearing produced a report on an inquiry into higher education and made recommendations regarding the development of skills seen as essential for all graduates to develop:

> we believe that four skills are key to the future success of graduates whatever they intend to do in later life. These four are: communication skills; numeracy; the use of information technology; learning how to learn.
>
> (Dearing, 1997, s9:17)

These key skills are now embedded in university programmes and will be part of the assessment criteria in your programme or module outlines. The primary focus of this book is to facilitate the development of students' use of information technology (IT), so they can efficiently access the quality information needed to support their studies and their practice. Using IT is often described as 'information literacy skills' and includes library skills, word-processing, data-management and the use of the internet and email.

However, information literacy skills cannot be seen in isolation from the other key transferable skills identified by Dearing (1997). In particular, communication and using IT are interdependent skills. Therefore, this first chapter will review aspects of these two key skills through the use of a series of self-assessment tools, to enable students to identify any areas that need further development before embarking on the more specific aspects of information literacy skills needed by nursing students.

Academic failure is one of the key factors influencing students leaving university (DH, 2007; Yorke and Longden, 2008). This chapter is designed to allow you to assess whether you have the necessary key skills to be successful at university, and to formulate a plan to further develop the skills you have and address any areas of weakness.

If you have studied recently and feel confident in your academic writing skills, go to the end of the chapter and complete the 'Knowledge review'. Once you have assessed your knowledge, you can decide which sections of this chapter you need to read or if you can safely move straight to Chapter 2.

For those who have not studied for a while, or are not confident in their academic ability, it will be useful to work though this chapter to identify key skills that need developing. Once areas for improvement have been identified, it is possible to make a plan for developing these skills and thus reducing the risk of academic failure. Effective preparation and awareness of the expectations of higher education are the keys to successful studying.

It is not only the university that sets standards for nursing students. The Nursing and Midwifery Council (NMC) has standards in terms of the knowledge and skills it expects nursing students to have at registration. The new standards are outlined in the 'Competency framework' of the draft *Standards for Pre-registration Nursing Education* (NMC, 2010). The boxes at the start of each chapter of this book show the specific learning skills that are relevant to each chapter and that the NMC expects you to have to be able to register as a nurse.

The NMC also expects nurses to continue to develop their knowledge and skills throughout their professional career, as specified in the NMC *Code* (2008a). This aspect will be considered in the section on personal development planning.

Communication skills

Communication involves both verbal and non-verbal skills, and includes verbal presentation and body language, as well as written and electronic communication. This chapter will focus primarily on verbal, written and electronic communication.

Verbal communication

When you are with your friends and family you will share a common language that enables you to feel confident to express your views and opinions freely. At university and in practice the language used will include words you are unfamiliar with and it may sometimes feel as if people are speaking a foreign language. This can result in you initially lacking the confidence to participate in discussions or ask questions when in the classroom and practice settings.

There are some things that may help you in this situation. Many programme documents and books will contain a glossary that explains the meanings of words or terms used. Clinical placements often have a list of terms and abbreviations for students so that they can understand the 'language' of the placement. Investing in a nursing or medical dictionary can also help with demystifying the language. Making use of such information and finding the confidence to ask the meanings of words you do not understand is vitally important. Asking questions is often seen as a sign of enthusiasm and interest and not as a negative attribute.

Practical tip

Buy yourself a small, pocket-sized address book that you can use to write down the meanings of new words you encounter. You can take this with you on practice placements until you are confident in the meanings of medical and nursing terms and abbreviations.

Communicating verbally is seen as an essential skill in nursing (NMC, 2007, 2008a) and is the vehicle through which respect, compassion and caring are communicated to patients/clients and relatives/carers. Non-verbal communication also plays an integral part in supporting the communication of these concepts.

Communication at university and in practice needs to be clear and concise, and delivered assertively to ensure that the message you wish to send is received correctly. Recent reports and research studies have identified communication failure as a central factor in cases where patients/clients suffer avoidable harm (Laming, 2003; NPSA, 2007), so developing a clear and confident communication style is a crucial aspect of professional practice.

Haig et al. (2006) propose the SBAR model for effectively communicating information in the health and social care context. This model takes account of the following factors.

- **Situation** – what is happening at the moment that warrants communication?
- **Background** – explain the circumstances leading up to this situation. Put the situation in context.
- **Assessment** – what do you think the problem is?
- **Recommendation** – what would you do to correct the problem?

Although designed for communication in practice, this model could also be used effectively in the university context when you have a need to communicate an issue to one of your tutors, or in everyday life as in the scenario below.

Scenario: Telephone conversation with the vet

Imagine your pet becomes ill and you need to telephone the vet to make an appointment. Below is an example of how you might use SBAR in an everyday situation.

Good morning . . .
Situation: My name is Jenny Smith and I need to make an appointment for my dog to be seen today by the vet, as he is limping badly and seems in a lot of pain in his right front leg.

Scenario continued

Background: Paddy is a five-year-old cocker spaniel and is registered with your surgery. He has never had anything like this before. We went for a long walk yesterday and he seemed fine yesterday evening.

Assessment: However, one of the pads on his right front paw seems tender to the touch and I wondered whether he may have picked up a grass seed or thorn on the walk and this is causing the problem.

Recommendation: I would like an appointment for him to be seen today as he is in so much pain.

Work through Activity 1.1 using the SBAR approach.

Activity 1.1   Communication

Think of a time when you have had to make a verbal complaint or enquiry. Perhaps something you have purchased has developed a fault and you needed to return the goods. Alternatively, you could think about a time when you needed to solve a problem. For example, you may have been feeling unwell and needed to make an appointment to see your GP.

- Using the SBAR model above as a guide, develop a *concise* verbal explanation of the situation, the context, your perspective on the problem and what you would like to happen. Remember to be assertive, not aggressive.
- Consider how closely this verbal communication compares with your actual experience. Has the model enabled you to be more concise and precise in your communication?

Try using this model in everyday situations where effective communication is particularly important. Repeated practice will make using SBAR second nature.

As this activity depends on your own experience, there is no outline answer at the end of the chapter.

Written communication

Good record keeping is viewed as 'an integral part of nursing' (NMC, 2009) and yet cases involving poor documentation of care are commonly brought before the NMC. Nurses also have a legal duty to maintain accurate records. Poor written communication has also been a contributory factor in many situations that have resulted in harm to the patient (NPSA, 2007). Poor documentation of care can lead to complaints being upheld and action being taken against nurses by the NMC and/or by the legal system. As you are a student, your mentor is accountable for all your patient documentation and will check and countersign all patient records you complete. However, you are responsible for your written records and it is essential that you are aware of the NMC requirements for nursing documentation and any additional NHS Trust policy relating to patient records.

The NMC (2009) outlines 16 principles for good record keeping (see box below). Although some of these principles are specific to record keeping, others are transferable to the principles underpinning academic writing, such as numbers 5, 6, 13 and 15.

Concept summary: NMC principles of good record keeping

1. Handwriting should be legible.
2. All entries to records should be signed. In the case of written records, the person's name and job title should be printed alongside the first entry.
3. In line with local policy, you should put the date and time on all records. This should be in real time and chronological order and be as close to the actual time as possible.
4. Your records should be accurate and recorded in such a way that the meaning is clear.
5. Records should be factual and not include unnecessary abbreviations, jargon, meaningless phrases or irrelevant speculation.
6. You should use your professional judgement to decide what is relevant and what should be recorded.
7. You should record details of any assessments and reviews undertaken and provide clear evidence of the arrangements you have made for future and ongoing care. This should also include details of information given about care and treatment.
8. Records should identify any risks or problems that have arisen and show the action taken to deal with them.
9. You have a duty to communicate fully and effectively with your colleagues, ensuring that they have all the information they need about the people in your care.
10. You must not alter or destroy any records without being authorised to do so.
11. In the unlikely event that you need to alter your own or another healthcare professional's records, you must give your name and job title, and sign and date the original documentation. You should make sure that the alterations you make, and the original record, are clear and auditable.
12. Where appropriate, the person in your care, or their carer, should be involved in the record keeping process.
13. The language that you use should be easily understood by the people in your care.
14. Records should be readable when photocopied or scanned.
15. You should not use coded expressions of sarcasm or humorous abbreviations to describe the people in your care.
16. You should not falsify records.

Source: NMC (2009, pp2–3).

Confidentiality and consent are other aspects of record keeping that also apply to academic work when examples from practice are used within academic assignments. However, there are additional factors that need to be taken into consideration when using written communication in academic work, which, if well developed, will also enhance record keeping in practice.

It is important that any written information conforms to grammatical and punctuation conventions. This does not just apply to academic work but is also an important aspect of record keeping. Patient records may well be reproduced in a court of law or disciplinary meeting, where errors of spelling, punctuation and expression may be highlighted as evidence of poor practice or may lead to alternative interpretations being made of your documentation that you did not intend.

Activity 1.2   Reflection

This activity is designed to enable you to assess your level of communication skills. Complete the table below and add up your scores before moving on to the next section.

	Please circle the number that applies	Not confident at all	Fairly confident	Confident	Very confident	Completely confident
A	How confident are you that your writing is legible?	0	1	2	3	4
B	How confident are you that your spelling, punctuation and grammar are good?	0	1	2	3	4
C	How confident are you that you can write a formal letter, explaining clearly its purpose?	0	1	2	3	4
D	How confident are you when making verbal enquiries?	0	1	2	3	4
E	How confident are you that you can verbally express yourself clearly and concisely?	0	1	2	3	4
F	How confident are you that you can be assertive when necessary?	0	1	2	3	4
	Total score					

Read on to assess your results.

Interpreting your score

If you scored 0 or 1 in any of the A–F categories, you need to focus on these areas just to ensure that your written and spoken English is of a good standard. If you scored poorly for B, a visit to the BBC Skillswise website (**www.bbc.co.uk/skillswise/words/grammar**) and working through some of the exercises there will help you to improve your use of English. You could also invest in a small pocket dictionary to check your spelling. Be careful when using the computer to check spelling or grammar, as these are not always accurate in the proposals they make for changes.

Feeling confident when speaking or explaining things to others may be more of a challenge. Improvement often only comes with practice and coaching. Take opportunities to participate in small group discussions in university and to explain things to your mentor while in practice. Listen to your mentor when he or she gives information to patients or is assertive with colleagues. This will help you to develop your own communication techniques.

If your score in each section is 2 or above, you have sufficient skills to begin your programme.

If you are unsure of your abilities in these basic writing skills, the next section will provide a helpful review of the essential rules. If you feel confident in your writing ability, you might just want to skim read this section.

Writing in sentences and paragraphs

It is extremely difficult to make sense of anything written in poorly constructed sentences. A sentence has three essential elements. First, it must make sense when read by itself; second, it must use correct punctuation; and, third, it must contain two kinds of words: a subject and a verb (doing word).

Activity 1.3	Communication

Which of the following is not a sentence, and why?

1. I walked to the shop.
2. In the trees.
3. The bus had left.
4. Wearing grey joggers.

There is an answer to this activity at the end of the chapter.

If you need to improve your sentence construction, the BBC Skillswise website mentioned above has very good information on grammar and punctuation. If you prefer face-to-face guidance, use your university study support centre if you are already a student, or try your local council adult education centre, as they may provide a free adult literacy service that may be more convenient.

In addition, it is important not to use overlong sentences as this often results in the meaning of the sentence being lost to the reader. Marks will be lost through unclear expression, so try to keep sentences to a maximum of two lines.

Paragraphing may seem unimportant to the student when writing an essay, but it is a very important aspect of any written communication as it indicates to the reader when discussion of one topic has been concluded and another topic begins. This provides structure to the written communication and allows arguments and discussions to be followed more easily.

The absence or incorrect use of punctuation also changes the meaning of a sentence. Take a look at the box below to see an example of this.

Concept summary: Sentence construction and punctuation

The book *Eats, Shoots and Leaves* (Truss, 2003) contains excellent examples of how punctuation alters the meaning of a sentence. The book title can be used as an example. Without punctuation the sentence is concerned with the diet of the animal, e.g. 'the panda eats shoots and leaves'.

Adding punctuation to the sentence alters the meaning, e.g. 'the panda eats, shoots and leaves'. This changes the meaning and sense of the sentence by suggesting that the panda eats something, then shoots someone or something and then leaves a place.

As you can see, sentence construction and punctuation are very important when writing information and ensuring that the correct meaning is conveyed. Use what you have learnt so far about communication to improve the letter in Activity 1.4.

Activity 1.4   *Communication*

Mark is concerned about the state of the pavement outside his home and decides to write to the council to complain and ask for action to be taken. Read his letter. Does it make sense?

> *Dear Sir,*
>
> *Will you please send someone to mend the pavement outside my house? My wife tripped and fell on it yesterday and now she is pregnant.*
>
> *Mark Jones*

Now rewrite this letter using SBAR (see page 6).

- **Situation** – what is happening at the moment that warrants communication?
- **Background** – explain the circumstances leading up to this situation. Put the situation in context.
- **Assessment** – what do you think the problem is?
- **Recommendation** – what would you do to correct the problem?

An example of a rewritten letter is given at the end of the chapter.

Before moving on to the next section, think about how the example letter at the end of this chapter compares with yours. How well did you use SBAR? Did you include all the relevant information that would enable the council to understand what had happened and what needed to be done? Remember that the more you practise using SBAR, the more effective your communication will be. Also think about whether your sentences were constructed well. Did they have a subject and a verb? Were they the right length? Was the punctuation correct? Did you use paragraphing appropriately?

Academic writing style

There are several elements that make writing academic. These include the writing style, wide reading evidenced by the use of references to support discussion, and the development of critical debate. Traditionally, academic essays are written in a formal writing style using the third person, in order to present an objective account of the topic under discussion. This involves avoiding the use of the first person 'I' or the second person 'we' or 'you', and instead writing in a more impersonal way. Note that the use of the words 'the author' or 'the student' instead of 'I' should be avoided as this does not change the sentence into the third person.

Initially, students often find this form of writing difficult. The scenario below illustrates how sentences written in the first person can be transformed into the third person.

Scenario: First person to third person

First person example

I noticed that the patient was in pain. When I asked the patient how he was, he said that he had severe pain in his back and wondered if he could have some pain killers.

Third person example

The patient's facial expression and body language suggested that he was experiencing severe pain. When the patient was questioned, he confirmed that he was experiencing extreme pain in his back and requested some analgesia.

Some lecturers would argue that writing in the third person also encourages the development of other academic writing skills. For example, it can lead to the use of literature and other evidence to demonstrate knowledge and understanding of the topic, and to develop critical debate through analysis and evaluation. The third person example above could be developed further through the introduction of some literature, as illustrated in the next scenario.

Scenario: Using references to literature

The patient's facial expression and body language suggested that he was experiencing severe pain. Burnard (2008) suggests that recognising and responding to non-verbal communication are essential aspects of the communication skills a nurse must develop in order to provide quality care. However, it is important to confirm with the patient verbally that the initial assumption, based on observation of non-verbal communication, is correct (Stringer, 2009). When the patient was questioned he confirmed that he was experiencing extreme pain in his back and requested some analgesia. This confirmed the initial perceptions and the patient was promptly provided with appropriate analgesia.

The last three sentences in the example illustrate how depth of discussion can be achieved by including references to additional literature and the integration of theory with practice experience. This could be achieved by writing in the first person, but care must be taken that, when written in the first person, the essay does not just become a descriptive story that will gain few marks.

Academic work is normally written in the third person, but this does not necessarily apply to reflective writing. It is therefore important to check assignment guidelines, or ask the programme or module leader whether they expect the assignment to be written in the first or third person to avoid being penalised.

Any academic piece of work demands support from the literature. This requires students to access, read and interpret information from a range of reliable sources, in order to ensure that they have the required depth of knowledge and understanding to meet the learning outcomes of the modules they are undertaking. This topic will be discussed further in Chapters 2 and 3.

Electronic communication

Emails, texting and using social networking sites such as Facebook are all examples of methods of communication developed in the digital age. This has led to an increase in the speed in which information can be communicated to the click of a button. Although this has its advantages, there are some disadvantages to these modes of communication.

In the same way that language may be used differently when speaking to friends and family than in formal situations such as the workplace, care must be taken to prevent informal texting language being used in emails to the university staff. You will need to communicate with your personal tutor, other lecturers and administrative staff during your time at university. Lecturers receive many emails every day from their students and it is important that simple conventions are observed.

1. Address the person you are emailing by name, e.g. Dear Jenny.
2. Use SBAR (see page 6) to clearly state what your email is about.
3. Do not use texting language in emails.

4. Make sure that any attachments *are* actually attached and are in a format that the tutor can open. (For example, if you use Microsoft Works at home to produce a document, your tutor may not be able to open it as most universities use Microsoft Word.)
5. End the email with your name.
6. Ensure that your signature information is completed on your email.

Below is an example of an email to a personal tutor.

Scenario: An appropriate email

Emma is a first-year student and needs to contact her personal tutor for an urgent appointment. She sends the quick email below.

Hay i need to see u i am off on tues so will c u then

A more appropriate email would be:

Dear Jenny,

I have an urgent problem I need to speak to you about. As you know I have been having some health problems and my GP has confirmed that I need urgent treatment. I am concerned how this will impact on my ability to attend place-ments. I could come to see you any time on Tuesday or at 5 p.m. on Wednesday. If neither of these times is convenient could you please phone me on my mobile: 077877777.

Thank you,

Emma Booth

S06, Child Nursing

Social networking

In 2008, the NMC issued the following statement:

The NMC would like to remind nurses and midwives that they are personally accountable for their actions at all times, including how they behave in their personal life.

(NMC, 2008b)

It goes on to make particular reference to Facebook:

Used properly, social networking sites such as Facebook are a great way to find old friends, join interest groups and share information. However, nurses and midwives should remember that anything posted on a social networking site is in the public domain.

What may be considered to be letting off steam about a situation at work can potentially be read by someone who may take offence at the content of a posting.

Nurses and midwives could be putting their registration at risk if posting inappropriate comments about colleagues or patients or posting any material that could be considered explicit.

(NMC, 2008b)

The NMC is not saying nurses should not use Facebook, but that they should do so responsibly and mindful of the fact that *The Code* (NMC, 2008a) applies to your private as well as your professional behaviour.

Numeracy skills

The NMC Essential Skills Cluster, Medicines management, clearly states that the newly qualified nurse *Accurately calculates medicines and ensures those responsible to the nurse are competent to do the same* (NMC, 2010, p105).

If you feel you need to revise your numeracy skills, speak to your personal tutor for guidance, or access one of the helpful books on the subject, such as *Passing Calculation Tests for Nursing Students*, also in the Transforming Nursing Practice series.

Using information technology

Information technology (IT) can seem far removed from caring for the patient at the bedside. However, the NMC clearly states that information management is an integral aspect of evidence-based practice, alongside the ability to access information from a range of sources. It is also widely acknowledged that IT is playing an increasingly important part in care provision. A visit to the NHS Connecting for Health website (**www.connectingforhealth.nhs.uk**) will illustrate the importance of computer skills in a modern health service. The move to providing more care in the community will increase the demand for information to be accessible electronically, allowing ease of access to patient data. Sound IT skills will be essential for anyone working in the NHS.

Students entering a nurse education programme will need some basic IT skills that include:

- using the internet/intranet to access patient information, or to find research and other literature to support practice, or for academic work, as well as for making referrals, record keeping and care planning;
- the ability to email and send attachments;
- word-processing skills to produce a Word document.

In addition, they will need to develop further skills during their programme that include:

- information literacy, to access a range of information sources in order to keep up to date;
- accessing learning resources via the university visual learning environment;
- using a PowerPoint presentation to convey information to others;
- using a spreadsheet to enter and manipulate data.

Complete Activity 1.5 to assess whether you need to work on any of the above areas.

Activity 1.5 — Reflection

	Please circle the number that applies	Not confident at all	Fairly confident	Confident	Very confident	Completely confident
A	How confident are you that you can create a word-processed document?	0	1	2	3	4
B	How confident are you that you can save, store and retrieve a word-processed document?	0	1	2	3	4
C	How confident are you that you can create and send an email?	0	1	2	3	4
D	How confident are you that you can create and send an email with an attachment?	0	1	2	3	4
E	How confident are you at using a library catalogue to find a book?	0	1	2	3	4
F	How confident are you that you can access a journal article on the internet?	0	1	2	3	4
G	How confident are you at using bibliographic databases or information gateways to find information to inform your practice?	0	1	2	3	4
H	How confident are you in accessing government and NHS websites to search for information?	0	1	2	3	4
	Total score					

Read on to assess your results.

Interpreting your scores

If you scored 8 or more in A–D, you have sound, basic IT skills on which to build. If you scored 4 or less in these sections, you will need to improve your computer skills before starting your university programme.

Sections E–H are more specific and represent the information literacy skills you will need to develop over the first few months of your programme. If your score in any of these sections is below 2, you will need to access the university study support and library services in order to improve these skills once you begin your programme.

Learning to learn

This section will consider other factors that you will need to think about when you attend university. Once there, you will only spend a proportion of the week attending lectures or seminars. The rest of the time you will be expected to study independently or with groups of other students. The temptation will be to see this un-timetabled time as 'free time' that you can use to socialise or to work to gain extra income. Although it is important to have fun and to keep your level of debt to a minimum, you will not succeed at university unless you make time to study.

You will be provided with a student handbook that you will be expected to read. Spending time reading the handbook will enable you to understand how much time you are expected to spend on your studies each week, and will help you to understand the rules and regulations of the university as well as your rights and expectations.

Managing your time

The university timetable will outline what days and times you will be expected to attend specific teaching and learning activities. You need to keep a record of this so that you can plan your activities around these dates and times. When you are attending university, plan in time to go to the library to study. Making effective use of your time during the week will free up time at the weekend for family and friends.

You will be expected to prepare for your sessions at university, for example by reading lecture notes or doing preparatory work with other students. In either case, these activities will require you to read and digest information before attending the university session. It is important to plan reading into your study week so that it becomes a habit. However, it is not advisable to set aside whole days for reading, as it will get more difficult to assimilate information as the day progresses. Break up the day, perhaps by building in some exercise such as walking or swimming, to help create some thinking space before returning to your reading.

Make use of smaller amounts of time for reading. For example, if you are an early riser, get up an hour earlier two or three mornings a week and use the time to read your notes or any articles and books that have been recommended, or to prepare for the week's lectures. Experiment to find out what your best time for studying is and then make sure you use this time effectively. It is important to give yourself time to assimilate what you have read before you need to use the information.

Accessing support systems

You will normally be allocated a personal tutor who will provide guidance and support for you during your studies, with the aim of promoting your academic development. He or she will advise you on how to develop your work in the light of feedback from your assignments, and will also provide support and guidance if personal or health issues interfere with your ability to study or attend placements.

Universities also provide a range of support services, from counselling to financial advice, through their student services unit. They are there to provide a confidential service for students, and personal tutors will not have access to any information regarding their students' use of this service.

The student union may also prove to be a useful source of advice and information on other aspects of your university life.

Personal development planning

Personal development planning (PDP) is a process that you will repeat at regular intervals during your nursing programme and in your professional life. It is a requirement of the NMC (2004, 2008a) and an expectation of professionals working within the NHS. Jasper (2006) suggests that professional development will continue throughout the working life of all professionals. Initially, your personal tutor and practice mentor will provide guidance in the development of your PDP until you become familiar with the process.

PDP often begins with a SWOT analysis:

- **S**trengths;
- **W**eaknesses;
- **O**pportunities;
- **T**hreats.

When used in a personal context, the SWOT analysis tool is designed to help develop your career by identifying your strengths and weakness, as well as the opportunities and threats that may enhance or impede your development (Mindtools, 2009). Having completed the learning activities in this chapter, the next step is to undertake a SWOT analysis.

Activity 1.6	*Reflection*

Take time to think about the strengths and weaknesses you have uncovered through undertaking the learning activities. Enter your strengths and weaknesses in the boxes below.

SWOT Analysis	
Strengths	Weaknesses
Opportunities	Threats

Once this is completed, consider what opportunities there are for you to build on your strengths and to eliminate your weaknesses. For example, you may be very confident in your ability to ask questions when you do not understand something, but have poor IT skills. Use your confidence and questioning ability to create an opportunity to gain access to IT training.

Opportunities are the third element of the SWOT analysis. IT training, library or study skills workshops could all be seen as opportunities to develop your key graduate skills. Make sure you make the most of them.

Finally, threats may be those things that get in the way of you improving your skills or gaining new ones. For example, if you do not have your own computer or internet access at home, your studies will be compromised. In this case it will be essential that you make full use of the time you are in university to access a computer and keep up with your work.

Having completed the analysis, the next step is to develop a personal development plan (PDP) to meet your learning needs.

A PDP is designed to *facilitate growth and development of an individual* (Evans, 2003, p3). It does this by identifying specific objectives aimed at addressing specific development needs and identifying any resources that may be needed to support that development.

In order to complete your PDP, you need to spend time clarifying your learning needs as identified in your self-assessments and SWOT analysis. When developing objectives it is useful to use the acronym SMART, so that the objectives you set yourself are: **s**pecific, **m**easurable, **a**chievable, **r**elevant and **t**ime-framed.

Table 1.1: SMART objectives

Specific	State exactly what you want to achieve	Example: Learn how to send an email with an attachment
Measurable	State how the objective will be measured so that you know when you have achieved your goal	Example: Can send an email attachment to my personal tutor
Achievable	Can the objective be achieved in the time-frame you have set? Are sufficient resources available?	Example: Booked into basic IT workshop in second week of term
Relevant	Will the achievement of the objective lead to desired results?	Example: Yes. I will be able to send work to my tutor by emailed attachment and receive feedback on my work
Time-framed	Set a date by which the objective will be achieved	Example: By the end of the third week of term

Below is a worked example of a PDP so you can see what this looks like in practice.

Personal Development Plan			20 September 2010
Specific objective	**How will I know when it is achieved?**	**What resources will I need?**	**When will this be achieved by?**
1. Make use of independent learning time for study	When I have created a weekly timetable and complete planned activities	Buy a diary and use to plan weekly study	25/9/10
2. Improve my email and internet skills	When I can confidently send an email without assistance	Attend basic IT workshop 30/9/10	5/10/10
3. Improve my library skills	When I can confidently find information using the university electronic resources such as CINAHL	Attend library workshop 14/10/10, 20/10/10 and 26/10/10	Library catalogue by 20/10/10 E-journals - 1/11/10 Bibliographic database 07/1/11

Taking responsibility for your own learning is the key to being successful in your studies at university. Creating a weekly timetable that makes good use of time for study and recreation, and making a clear PDP, are two steps you can take towards becoming an effective learner.

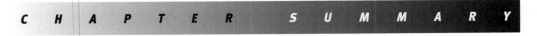

CHAPTER SUMMARY

This chapter has introduced you to the key graduate skills needed to be successful at university and in your professional practice as a nurse. It has provided you with the opportunity to assess your own key skills using a range of self-assessment activities, and to undertake a SWOT analysis. You have been introduced to the concept of personal development planning (PDP) and encouraged to use the outcomes of the SWOT analysis to create a PDP for future learning using SMART objectives.

Check how much you have learnt

Undertake the following short test to see how much you have learnt by completing this chapter. Answers are provided below.

1. List Dearing's four key skills.
    i.
    ii.
    iii.
    iv.

2. Draw a line between each element of the SBAR model and the correct description.

Elements		Description
S		What do you think the problem is?
B		What is happening at the moment that warrants communication?
A		What would you do to correct the problem?
R		Explain the circumstances leading up to the situation. Put the situation in context.

3. Give four reasons why IT skills are needed by nurses.
    i.
    ii.
    iii.
    iv.

4. What does SWOT stand for?
   S
   W
   O
   T

5. Give three reasons why it is important to create your own university timetable.
   i.
   ii.
   iii.

6. What are SMART objectives?
   S
   M
   A
   R
   T

Answers

1. Dearing's four key skills are:
   i.   communication skills;
   ii.   numeracy;
   iii. use of information technology;
   iv.   learning how to learn.

2. The correct descriptions in the SBAR model of communication are as follows.

Elements	Description
S	What is happening at the moment that warrants communication?
B	Explain the circumstances leading up to the situation. Put the situation in context.
A	What do you think the problem is?
R	What would you do to correct the problem?

3. Four reasons why IT skills are needed by nurses are:
   i.   to access patient-related and professional information, e.g. on the internet/intranet;
   ii.   to communicate with colleagues and other professionals, e.g. by email;
   iii. to prepare reports and patient records, e.g. by using word-processing skills;
   iv.   to communicate and share information with colleagues, e.g. by using presentation skills.

4. SWOT stands for:
   Strengths;
   Weaknesses;
   Opportunities;
   Threats.

5. It is important to create your own university timetable:
   i.   to make the best use of your study time;
   ii. to build in time for reading, study and recreation;
   iii. to take responsibility for your own learning.
6. The SMART objectives are:
   Smart;
   Measurable;
   Achievable;
   Realistic;
   Timely.

Activities: brief outline answers

Activity 1.3: Communication (page 10)

1. This is a complete sentence. It makes sense. It has a subject 'I' and a verb 'walked'.
2. This sentence is incomplete as it does not make sense on its own and has no subject or verb. Adding these would make it a complete sentence, e.g. The birds were singing in the trees.
3. This sentence is complete as it has a subject and a verb.
4. This sentence is incomplete as it is missing the subject. By adding a subject the sentence makes sense, e.g. The boy was wearing grey joggers.

Activity 1.4: Communication (page 11)

Dear Sir,

S
We live at 22 Station Road, Barming, and we are expecting our first baby in two months. Yesterday my wife fell heavily on the pavement outside our front gate and badly twisted her ankle.

B
The pavement outside our home is in a poor condition. Some of the paving slabs are cracked and the surface is very uneven. I reported this to your highways department on two previous occasions: March 1st by letter and May 5th by telephone. I have had no reply to indicate what action you intend to take to repair the pavement.

A
We were very concerned that the fall may have harmed the baby or resulted in my wife going into premature labour. The injury to her ankle has caused her considerable pain and discomfort, and required attendance at our local accident and emergency department. I believe that, had the repairs to the pavement been undertaken when requested, my wife would not have fallen.

R
There is now an urgent need to repair the pavement to prevent another accident happening. I anticipate an early response to this letter.

Yours sincerely,
Mark Jones

Knowledge review

Having completed the chapter, how would you now rate your knowledge of the following topics?

	Good	Adequate	Poor
1. Dearing's key skills.			
2. Communication skills.			
3. Academic writing.			
4. Using information technology.			
5. Learning to learn.			

Where you're not confident in your knowledge of a topic, what will you do next?

Further reading

For further information on academic writing:
Cottrell, S (2008) *The Study Skills Handbook*, 3rd edn. Basingstoke: Palgrave Macmillan.
Price, B and Harrington, A (2010) *Critical Thinking and Writing for Nursing Students.* Exeter: Learning Matters.
Rose, J (2007) *The Mature Student's Guide to Writing*, 2nd edn. Basingstoke: Palgrave Macmillan.

For further information on communication:
Bach, S and Grant, A (2009) *Communication and Interpersonal Skills for Nurses.* Exeter: Learning Matters.
Stein-Parbury, J (2009) *Patient and Person: Interpersonal skills in nursing*, 4th edn. Chatswood, NSW: Elsevier.

For further information on numeracy:
Lapham, R (2009) *Drug Calculations for Nurses: A step-by-step approach*, 2nd edn. London: Arnold.
Starkings, S and Krause, L (2010) *Passing Calculations Tests for Nursing Students.* Exeter: Learning Matters.

For further information on personal development planning (PDP):
Cottrell, S (2003) *Skills for Success.* Basingstoke: Palgrave Macmillan.
Jasper, M (2006) *Reflection, Decision-making and Professional Development.* Oxford: Blackwell.

Useful websites

www.businessballs.com/swotanalysisfreetemplate.htm Businessballs – to learn more about using a SWOT analysis.
www.mindtools.com/pages/article/newTMC_05.htm Mindtools – also to learn more about using a SWOT analysis.
www.skills4study.com Palgrave Study Skills – a free resource full of practical advice to help you study more effectively at university.

Chapter 2

Planning a search for information

Draft NMC Standards for Pre-registration Nursing Education

This chapter will address the following draft competencies:

Domain: Professional values

8. All nurses must be responsible and accountable for keeping their own knowledge and skills up-to-date through continuing professional development and life-long learning. They must use evaluation, supervision and appraisal to improve their performance and enhance the safety and quality of care and service delivery.

Domain: Nursing practice and decision making

6. All nurses must use a range of information and data to improve the health of individuals, communities and populations, and support decision making. They must help people and their carers make choices about their health care needs.
9. All nurses must use up-to-date knowledge to decide the best way to deliver safe, evidence-based care across all ages.
10. All nurses must use their knowledge of research and current nursing and associated knowledge to evaluate care, communicate findings, influence change and promote best practice.

Draft Essential Skills Clusters

Cluster: Organisational aspects of care

10. People can trust the newly registered graduate nurse to deliver nursing interventions and evaluate their effectiveness against the agreed assessment and care plan.

By the second progression point:

iv. Actively seeks to extend knowledge and skills using a variety of methods in order to enhance care delivery.

15. People can trust the newly registered graduate nurse to safely delegate to others and to respond appropriately when a task is delegated to them.

By entry to the register:

v. Recognises and addresses deficits in knowledge and skill in self and others and takes appropriate action.

QAA Subject benchmark statements

ClC2 Skills

Information gathering

The award holder should be able to demonstrate:

- an ability to gather and evaluate evidence and information from a wide range of sources;
- an ability to use methods of enquiry to collect and interpret data in order to provide information that would inform or benefit practice.

Information technology

The award holder should be able to demonstrate:

- an ability to engage with technology, particularly the effective and efficient use of information and communication technology.

Chapter aims

After reading this chapter, you will be able to:

- create a plan for a search for information;
- understand how Boolean operators can be used to refine or expand a search for information;
- appreciate the limitations of searching on the internet;
- understand the importance of keeping accurate records when searching the internet.

Introduction

Nurses are required to provide the best quality care possible for the people seeking help or support for their healthcare needs. To do this they are expected to be aware of current research, policies, standards, guidance and recommendations for their area of professional practice, so that the care they provide is 'evidence-based'. This chapter has been designed to enable nursing students to develop the skills needed to search for, find and begin to evaluate the evidence that supports best professional practice and their university studies.

This chapter will outline how to develop and implement a search strategy. It will discuss the various sources/resources that can be used to access reliable information and will provide some frameworks for judging the quality of the information found.

Formulating a search strategy

When searching for information, particularly on the internet, it is very easy to become confused by and lost among the enormous amount of material available. It can also be very time-consuming and so use up more time than planned. Spending a little time planning your search for information at the beginning is likely to result in you being more successful at finding relevant information, thus saving you time in the long run.

Another consideration is the amount of time you will have to find information for your university assignments, as this will be limited by the assignment submission date, so good planning can help you make the most of the available study time. A well-planned search will also reduce the likelihood of you being sidetracked, looking at information that may only be distantly connected to your topic.

A strategy is simply a plan of action that uses particular approaches to ensure success. A search strategy requires six elements to be successful:

- selecting a topic;
- identification of key words (which words best describe your topic);
- focusing for your search;
- extending or refining your search;
- using appropriate sources;
- keeping a record of your search.

Step 1: Identification of key words

Key words are similar to the words you might find in the index of a book. In your textbooks the authors have provided you with the index so you can easily locate the precise piece of information you need using a key word. For example, you have a nursing textbook and may want some information on communication skills. Looking for the key word 'communication' in the index you are likely to find some information on the topic. However, you may also find relevant information under the key words 'interpersonal skills'. It is important to take time to think about other key words that may have the same or similar meaning, so that you do not miss important information stored under a different key word.

When searching the internet (or world wide web – www), the 'index' of key words will be vast. For example, entering 'communication' into the commercial search engine Google™ will result in excess of 260 million hits, which is an impossible amount of material to read through to find the specific communication information you are seeking. This would suggest that, if you want to find information on the internet, you need to be as specific with your key words as possible to reduce the number of hits to a manageable number.

Identifying key words may be a quick and simple task if the topic is one with which you are familiar. Taking five minutes to jot down single words associated with the topic may be all that is needed for you to produce a comprehensive list of key words. However, if the topic is new and unfamiliar to you, the task of identifying key words may be more of a challenge. In this situation you could begin by reading through course information or recommended literature in your module/programme bibliographies to help you identify key words. Alternatively, you can use a thesaurus, such as the one available at **www.thesaurus.com**. By entering your initial key word into this online thesaurus can help to expand your list of key words and increase the chances of finding relevant material. Using some of these ideas should not only enable you to increase your list of key words, but also to identify some key words that have the same or similar meanings.

At this early stage of a search, other internet sources can also be useful to expand the number of key words. Wikipedia, for example, is a free online encyclopaedia that can prove a useful starting point for identifying additional key words. Returning to our example of communication, Wikipedia provides a section on communication that includes definitions and is subdivided under content headings. However, Wikipedia should be used with caution in relation to academic work and professional practice. This issue will be discussed and explored further in Chapter 3 under the section on sources of information. However, as an initial source of information and key words on a topic Wikipedia can be very useful.

Having identified a number of key words, it is now possible to construct a spider diagram or mind map that enables you to identify the breadth of a topic. However, in undergraduate studies written assignments will be limited to between 1,500 and 5,000 words, and there will be an expectation that students will focus on a particular aspect of practice or study. Therefore, the next stage of the process is to begin to group key words under headings to focus the search activity. Figure 2.1 shows an example of a mind map of the key words associated with a search on the topic of abuse. This topic has relevance to all branches of nursing and midwifery.

Step 2: Focusing your search

Figure 2.1 identifies some of the areas that may be associated with the word 'abuse' and illustrates the broad nature of the topic. Any search would need to use the key word 'abuse' along with a combination of other key words to give the search a specific focus or to answer a specific question. It could be suggested that all professionals working in health and social care should have a sound understanding of their professional and legal responsibilities (shaded areas) in the context of abuse. However, from a profession-specific view, it is at this point that you will need to decide which aspect of the topic is most relevant to you in terms of what exactly it is you want to find out.

For example, adult nurses and children's nurses may wish to explore the area of diagnosis, prevention, professional accountability and the law. These nurses will meet many clients in the course of their professional work, and may notice that a patient has

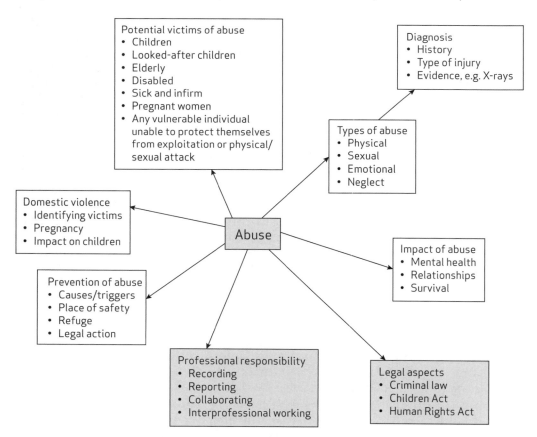

Figure 2.1: An initial mind map of key words on the topic of abuse

an unusual or unexplained injury, or perhaps a patient may appear frightened or unusually nervous in the company of a member of his or her family or a carer. All professionals need to be aware of the processes and procedures they are expected to undertake if they suspect a person has been a victim of abuse or neglect, the records they need to make about their concerns, and the referral processes. Adult and child protection has become an increasingly important focus in the health and social care context.

Mental health and learning disability nurses may have more interest in the impact of abuse on the mental health of the victim or the perpetrator, potential treatments, therapies and services available. However, the mentally ill or those with learning disabilities can also become the victims of abuse or exploitation, and so perhaps issues such as whistle blowing and accountability, consent and restraint may be added as key words to the search for these professional groups.

Midwives may have a particular interest in domestic violence and the evidence that the risk of violence increases when women become pregnant. Again, the law and professional recommendations and accountability will be areas in which midwives will need to develop a comprehensive understanding from the material they find. However, they will also need specific evidence to support the link between pregnancy and the potential for the expectant mother to experience increased domestic violence.

Once you have decided which area of the topic you are going to develop, you are then in a position to create a more focused list of key words to use in your search. These can also be used to develop search statements that can help with refining your search.

Step 3: Extending or refining your search

Once you have produced a number of key words relevant to your search, you need to consider how these might be combined to refine your search further when you are using electronic sources, for example commercial search engines, information gateways, library catalogues or databases. The words **AND** and **OR** are most commonly used for this process. These words (AND/OR) are called 'Boolean operators' and are named after the mathematician, George Boole.

Concept summary: Boolean operators

- **AND** allows you to **limit** your search for information to two or more subjects by developing search statements. For example, if you want to search on the physical abuse of children, your key words would be abuse, physical and children and would be combined using AND, e.g. abuse AND physical AND children. The search results will include only results that include the three key words.
- **OR** allows you to **broaden** your search for information where several different terms may be used for the same thing, e.g. elderly OR elder OR older person OR pensioner. By using all these terms a wider range of material can be accessed that relates to the elderly. By inserting the word OR, the search will ensure that the information found is about all the key words entered, but in this case not all the material found will include all the key words used.
- **NOT** is another Boolean operator that can be used to **limit** a search. For example, you may want to find information about 'abuse' and 'neglect' but find a lot of information on physical abuse is included. To refine your search you could add: NOT physical. This would exclude this term from your search if your main interest is neglect.

Concept summary continued

Not all search engines have the facility to refine searches in this way, so reducing the number of hits to a manageable number may not be easy or possible. Some bibliographic databases use the Boolean principle by allowing you to search for individual key words and then combining these searches to produce a smaller number of hits. These more sophisticated sources often allow you to further limit your search by year of publication or by the use of subheadings (e.g. CINAHL). This allows more precise searching.

Before starting to search for information it is important to identify which key words can be combined together to form search statements. You need to avoid typing long sentences into search engines, as this is likely to result in the inclusion of irrelevant material.

You need to think of your key words as a pyramid of words with the most precise terms at the apex of the pyramid and the broader terms at the bottom. For example, imagine you have been asked to find information on the topic of abuse as it relates to older people. If we return to our example of abuse and focus on abuse of the elderly our pyramid of words might look something like Figure 2.2.

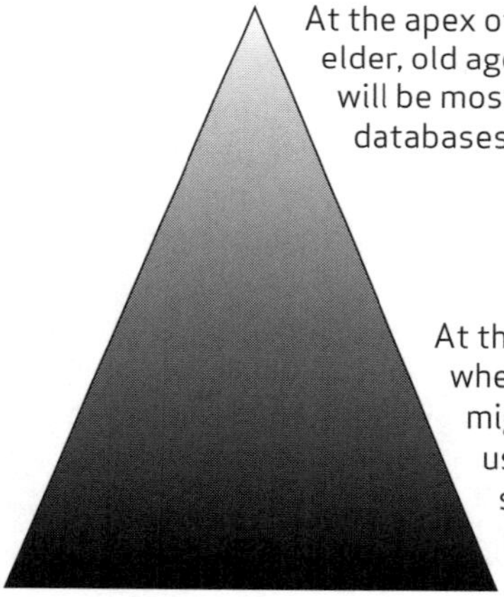

At the apex of the pyramid would be very precise key words, such as elderly, elder, old age and aged, alongside the main key word 'abuse'. These terms will be most useful when searching for journal articles in bibliographic databases.

At the base of the pyramid are broader terms that can be used when searching the library catalogue to find textbooks that might contain a chapter or section on elderly abuse. Key words used here might include 'elderly care' and very broad terms such as 'nursing care'. The book index and contents page would then be used to find the specific section on elderly abuse or adult protection.

Figure 2.2: Key word pyramid

Activity 2.1   *Research*

Use the suggestions in Figure 2.2 and the information on Boolean operators in the last Concept summary to create a list of search statements that could be used in an initial search for information on abuse of the elderly.

Compare your statements with the answer at the end of the chapter.

How did you get on? Did you manage to include all the other words that mean the same or are similar to 'elderly'? Don't worry if you found this task difficult. It takes practice.

If you decide to use two words together without AND or OR, it is useful to put them into double quotation marks as the search engine will then search for the words together rather than as a group of single words, for example 'elderly abuse'.

As you conduct your initial search you will begin to identify other key words that will help you to refine your search further. If you have found a particularly useful article, look to see if it has a list of key words on the first page. These will be the key words used to categorise the article in a bibliographic database, so it can be useful to check to see whether the article identifies any key words that are not on your list, but may help you to find other relevant articles.

You then need to decide on a focus for your search. For example, you may decide to focus on ways of detecting and preventing abuse and so add these key words to your search of the literature you have found. In this way your search becomes more organised and precise, and will find literature that can provide answers to specific questions, for example 'How can elderly abuse be prevented?', rather than being a random search on abuse of the elderly, which will produce too many hits for you to manage, as well as material that is irrelevant to your focus.

Step 4: Using appropriate sources

Having developed your key words and some search statements, you need to think about where you are going to look for information.

Activity 2.2   *Reflection and research*

- Imagine that you are planning a holiday. Take a few minutes to make a list of all the possible places you could go to gain information about possible holiday destinations.
- Once you have completed your list, make a second list that includes the things you will need to consider before you book your holiday.

Read on for comments on this activity.

When making your first list in Activity 2.2 it is likely that you identified resources such as travel agents, holiday brochures and websites. You may also have included websites that specialise in producing independent holiday reviews in order to check out the views of other holiday makers who have holidayed at your proposed destination before you book.

When choosing a holiday, people tend to 'shop around' to try to get the best value for money, so they look at a range of sources of information before making a decision. The same will be demanded of you in your nursing studies. You will be expected to read information from a range of sources in order for you to be confident that you have all the information you need to make decisions about the best evidence to support your practice and your academic studies.

In your second list, you will probably have included considerations such as cost, availability and time. Your university or college will provide you with access to a range of resources without charge, so it is important that you discover what these are and how to access them so you do not incur unnecessary costs by paying for resources you could access for free. For example, knowing your library account user name and password (formerly called ATHENS) will enable you to gain free access to the full text of articles online from those journals your library subscribes to. Your faculty/school librarian will provide advice on how to access your ATHENS account, as well as information on the resources available.

Choosing the right places to look for information

The resources available through your university library will generally be the most reliable and will have been recommended by academic staff as appropriate for your programme. Making decisions about the reliability of other sources you regularly have access to is an important skill to develop.

You will be familiar with finding information from a range of sources, such as newspapers, radio, television news and documentaries, or by searching the internet using commercial search engines like Google. However, you will need to learn about new resources when you join a nursing programme. This will take time and effort, but will benefit you by enabling you to access sources of information that you will use throughout your university studies and professional career.

This does not mean that you cannot use commercial search engines, blogs or Wikipedia to support your studies, but they do need to be used with caution. This is because anyone can publish on the internet, so it is possible that some material may be inaccurate, out of date or even deliberately misleading. When using these sources care must be taken to consider the following issues.

- Can you identify the author of the information?
- What qualifications do they have and can you find any other information about them on the internet that would confirm they are an expert in the field they are writing about?
- When was the material written? This is often difficult to establish on many websites.
- What evidence do they provide to support any statements or claims?
- What type of website is the information on? Is it a commercial site that is trying to encourage you to spend money on their products or is it a non-profit-making organisation such as a charity?
- Is it an academic website produced by a university or other academic institution?

In order to establish the type of website you are accessing, you need to be familiar with the information available from the URL (Uniform Resource Locator), which is often known as the web address.

As an example, look at elements of the URL for Google: **www.google.co.uk**. This is the domain name and it has several elements.

- www   =   world wide web (not all sites have this).
- google. =   Google is the name of the organisation that has exclusive rights to use that domain name.
- co.   =   This part of the domain tells you what type of organisation is publishing the website.
- .uk   =   This element tells you it is a UK-based website. (American websites often omit this element of the URL.)

From the example above we can see that this site is a version of the Google search engine offering UK-specific pages as well as world results. When considering this type of organisation, the fact that it is appended .co indicates that it is a commercial organ-isation. This suggests that the site is advertising or selling a product or service and so may not necessarily provide unbiased information.

In addition, anyone can publish on Google and there is no monitoring of content. As a consequence, information found through Google has to be viewed with caution and the questions listed above must be used to determine the reliability of the information accessed.

However, using Google can lead you to more reliable sites, such as government (.gov), NHS (.nhs) and academic (.ac) sites. If you are able to recognise the nature of the website you have accessed, you will be able to begin to make a judgement on the reliability of the material you have found on the site.

Wikis, blogs, Twitter and so on are increasingly popular, but as sources of information to enlighten university studies and professional practice, they must be viewed with caution as the reliability and accuracy of their content cannot be guaranteed. Blogs written by patients or carers can be very useful in providing individual perspectives, but cannot be generalised to reflect the views of all patients or carers in similar circumstances.

Activity 2.3	Research and critical thinking

Using a topic from your nursing studies, undertake a quick search on Google. Look at the URLs of the websites found in the first few pages of results. The majority are likely to be .co or .com. Think about how you might use the criteria listed on page 30 to judge whether the material is likely to be reliable enough to use in your studies or to support your clinical practice.

As this activity is based on your own nursing topic, there is no outline answer at the end of the chapter.

One feature of searching the internet is that it is sometimes difficult to find useful websites a second time. This is usually because no record was kept of the web address or the key words used to find the site. This can be annoying, but when using information to support professional practice and university studies, it becomes more significant as you will be expected to provide a reference for any source of information you use. This makes keeping a record of your searches really important.

Step 5: Keeping a record of your search

Now that you have developed a search strategy, you are ready to implement your plan, but before you begin there is one more task to consider, and that is keeping a record of your search. Keeping a record of *what* key words you used, *when* and *where* you have used them, and *what* information you found is an essential part of any search for information. Keeping accurate records of your search will save you a great deal of time and avoid the frustration of losing references to useful information.

Some electronic sources will allow you to save and/or print a record of your search, so take advantage of this facility where it exists. For other sources you may need to make a written record. You could use a simple framework, such as the one in Table 2.1.

This record does not have to be handwritten and there are electronic ways in which you can save the information you have found that will be explored in Chapter 6. The important fact is that you keep a record of your search and the reference details of what you found so that you do not waste your time searching for material that you have lost because of poor recording of results.

Table 2.2 shows a sample search diary that you can use to keep a record of your key words, search statements and resources used.

Table 2.1: Framework for an internet search

Key word(s)/ Statements	Source used and date accessed	Number of hits	Information accessed (e.g. full reference of articles and/or websites accessed)	Notes, e.g. how search was refined and any specific problems encountered
Abuse	Google 4/2/08	384,000,000	http://www.childline.org.uk/Childabuse.asp too much info., just accessed this website	No limits set; too much info. to sort through so just accessed childline website
Preventing abuse	Google 4/2/08	67,000	http://www.nspcc.org.uk/whatwedo/ whatwedohubpage_wda33342.html	Limited to UK only; first page of results not useful but found NSPCC site for background information
Abuse	CINAHL	4194	Saved search on pen drive in PD1 folder as need help from librarian to access full text articles; abstracts suggest several useful articles here	Original search reduced to 344 by restricting to 2007
Children	ASSIA	3739		
Physical	4/02/08	Reduced to 344		

Table 2.2: Developing a search strategy

Chosen topic:		
Mind map of key words on topic		Specific key words

Search statements using AND/OR		Sources to be used

Table 2.2: Continued

Key word(s)/ Statements	Source used and date accessed	Number of hits	Information accessed (e.g. full reference of articles and/or websites accessed)	Notes, e.g. how search was refined and any specific problems encountered

CHAPTER SUMMARY

This chapter has outlined how to develop a simple plan for finding information to inform your studies and your practice. It has covered the following aspects:

- identification of key words;
- extending or refining your search;
- focusing your search;
- keeping a record of your search.

Check how much you have learnt

Undertake the following short test to see how much you have learnt by completing this chapter. Answers are provided below.

1. List three reasons why planning your search can be an advantage.
   i.
   ii.
   iii.
2. Which type of statement/key word is most likely to help you find information on a topic in online journals? Tick the answer you think is correct.

   ❏   ❏

   Broad statement/key word   or   Specific statement/key word

   Why is this so? ....
   ....
   ....

3. Boolean operators help refine or expand a search. Draw a line between each Boolean operator and the correct answer.

Boolean operator		Answers
AND		Excludes certain terms from the search
OR		Limits the search to two or more keywords
NOT		Expands the search to include a range of similar terms

4. What does URL stand for?
   U
   R
   L

5. What do the following endings to a URL tell you about the organisation? Draw a line between each term on the left and the correct answer in the right-hand column.

Ending		Answer
.co or .com		A not-for-profit organisation such as a charity or carers' group
.ac		An NHS site that should contain reliable information relating to a specific service
.gov		An academic institution such as a university or college
.nhs		A commercial organisation that may be selling or advertising a product or service
.org		A government site that should contain reliable information relating to policy, laws, standards and guidelines etc.

6. Which of the above is most likely to contain unreliable information?

....

7. Why is it important that you keep a record of the source of the information you have found?

....

Answers

1. Three main reasons why planning your search can be an advantage are:
   i.   it saves time;
   ii. you are more likely to find the information you need;
   iii. you are less likely to find irrelevant information.
2. You should have ticked the right-hand box. The type of statement/key word that is most likely to help you find information on a topic in online journals is *specific*.

   Your reasons for why this is so should have included:
   - because journal databases contain key words in an index, so the more precise you are in the terms you use the more likely you are to find relevant material;
   - broad statements are better for searching library catalogues for book titles; you would then use specific terms to search the index of the book.
3. The Boolean operators and their correct functions are as follows.

Boolean operator	Answer
AND	Limits the search to two or more keywords
OR	Expands the search to include a range of similar terms
NOT	Excludes certain terms from the search

4. URL stands for:
   Uniform
   Resource
   Locator.
5. The URL endings and their correct meanings are as follows.

Ending	Answer
.co or .com	A commercial organisation that may be selling or advertising a product or service
.ac	An academic institution such as a university or college
.gov	A government site that should contain reliable information relating to policy, laws, standards and guidelines etc.
.nhs	An NHS site that should contain reliable information relating to a specific service
.org	A not-for-profit organisation such as a charity or carers' group

6. The URL element most likely to contain unreliable information is **.co** or **.com**.
7. The reasons why it is important that you keep a record of the sources of the information you have found are:
   - so that you can find the information again;
   - so that you can share what you have found with others;
   - so that you can use the sources as references in your university work;
   - so that you can justify your actions in practice;
   - to avoid plagiarism.

Activities: Brief outline answers

Activity 2.1: Research (page 28)

At the top of your pyramid (see Figure 2.2) could be the following *precise statements* (for use in bibliographic databases):

- elderly OR elder OR old age OR aged AND abuse;
- detecting AND preventing.

At the bottom of your pyramid could be the following *broad statements* (for searching in the library catalogue):

- nursing care;
- elderly care;
- geriatric care;
- nursing ethics.

Knowledge review

Having completed the chapter, how would you now rate your knowledge of the following topics?

	Good	Adequate	Poor
1. Planning a search.			
2. Refining/expanding your search using Boolean operators.			
3. URLs.			
4. Why material on the internet is not always reliable.			
5. Undertaking simple searches.			
6. Keeping a record of your search.			

Where you're not confident in your knowledge of a topic, what will you do next?

Further reading

Clark, A (2008) *E-Learning Skills*. Basingstoke: Palgrave Macmillan.
Pages 74–85 of this book have useful sections on searching for information and evaluating sources.

Cowen, M, Maier, P and Price, G (2009) *Study Skills for Nursing and Healthcare Students*. Harlow: Pearson Education.
Chapter 18 on using evidence-based practice has some useful guidance on undertaking a search for information.

Useful websites

www.brookes.ac.uk/library/webeval.html Oxford Brookes University: Evaluating web sources.
This site offers clear information for students trying to make judgements on sources of information on the internet.

www.vts.intute.ac.uk/ Virtual Training Suite, Intute.
This academic website offers a set of excellent online tutorials designed to help students improve their internet information skills. It offers subject-specific guidance and there is a section specifically for nurses.

Chapter 3

Going to the right places
for information

Draft NMC Standards for Pre-registration Nursing Education

This chapter will address the following draft competencies:

Domain: Professional values

8. All nurses must be responsible for keeping their own knowledge and skills up-to-date through continuing professional development and life-long learning. They must use evaluation, supervision and appraisal to improve their performance and enhance the safety and quality of care and service delivery.

Domain: Nursing practice and decision making

6. All nurses must use a range of information and data to improve the health of individuals, communities and populations, and support decision making. They must help people and their carers make choices about their health care needs.

9. All nurses must use up-to-date knowledge to decide the best way to deliver safe, evidence-based care across all ages.

10. All nurses must use their knowledge of research and current nursing and associated knowledge to evaluate care, communicate findings, influence change and promote best practice.

Domain: Leadership, management and team working

10. All nurses must draw on a range of resources to evaluate and audit care, and then use this information to contribute to improving people's experience and outcomes of care and the shaping of future services.

Draft Essential Skills Clusters

This chapter will address the following draft ESCs:

Cluster: Care, compassion and communication

1. As partners in the care process, people can trust a newly registered graduate nurse to provide collaborative care based on the highest standards, knowledge and competence.

Draft Essential Skills Clusters continued

By entry to the register:

viii. Demonstrates clinical confidence through sound knowledge, skills and understanding relevant to field.

Cluster: Organisational aspects of care

10. People can trust the newly registered graduate nurse to deliver nursing interventions and evaluate their effectiveness against the agreed assessment and care plan.

By the second progression point:

iv. Actively seeks to extend knowledge and skills using a variety of methods in order to enhance care delivery.

By entry to the register:

v. Recognises and addresses deficits in knowledge and skill in self and others and takes appropriate action.

QAA Subject benchmark statements

ClC2 Skills

Information gathering

The award holder should be able to demonstrate:
- an ability to gather and evaluate evidence and information from a wide range of sources.

Chapter aims

After reading this chapter, you will be able to:

- identify the various types of evidence that can be used to support practice;
- identify a range of reliable sources of information from which evidence can be accessed and used to inform your practice and educational studies.

Introduction

If you were looking for ideas and information on where to go on holiday, it seems obvious to state that you would seek these from a travel agent or holiday website and not from a company that sells suitcases. However, students sometimes struggle to find information relevant to their studies because they do not look in the right places for their particular subject. This chapter aims to provide sufficient guidance about a range of electronic sources to enable you to select the most appropriate sources for your studies. The chapter will begin with a discussion on what constitutes evidence before considering some of the available sources.

What constitutes evidence and where can it be accessed?

This section will begin by examining what is meant by the word 'evidence'. In the past research, particularly the randomised controlled trial, was seen as the evidence that should support practice. However, today the term 'evidence' has been broadened to encompass a wider range of information. This chapter will explore the nature of evidence and the status that evidence has in terms of traditional views of research. It will also outline some of the sources that can be used to identify specific types of evidence.

Traditional views of science and research suggest that there are two types of recognised research evidence: original studies based on experiment or observation (primary research); and reviews of published research that synthesise and combine findings using a systematic approach (secondary research) (University of Sheffield, 2010). This type of research evidence is often ranked in a hierarchy as outlined below, with 1 being the best and 7 being the least reliable to support practice (University of Sheffield, 2010).

1. Systematic reviews and meta-analysis.
2. Randomised controlled trials.
3. Cohort studies.
4. Cross-sectional surveys.
5. Case reports.
6. Expert opinion.
7. Anecdotal evidence.

Rycroft-Malone et al. (2004) offer an alternative perspective on what counts as evidence, and suggest that a broader interpretation is needed in order to deliver person-centred care. They propose four types of evidence that reflect the bringing together of the external (scientific) and the internal (intuitive) approaches to care. The four areas are:

- research;
- clinical experience;
- patient experience;
- information from the local context.

Table 3.1 illustrates how merging the traditional and more recent views of evidence places the more subjective and individual evidence at the lower end of the evidence hierarchy. However, it could be argued that, in order to provide person-focused care, there needs to be recognition of the value of other forms of evidence that can inform practice.

Table 3.1: Range of evidence and its sources

Traditional research hierarchy	Broader view of evidence	Examples of potential sources
1. Systematic reviews and meta-analysis	Research studies using a range of methodologies	Cochrane Library Bibliographic databases
2. Randomised controlled trials		Professional journals and periodicals NICE guidelines
3. Cohort studies		Professional journals and periodicals Office of National Statistics
4. Cross-sectional surveys	Information from local context, e.g. audit and case review	Information gateways, Department of Health, National Service Frameworks
5. Case reports		National Patient Safety Agency
6. Expert opinion	Clinical experience Patient experience	Professional journals and periodicals Newspapers and television
7. Anecdotal evidence	Clinical experience Patient experience	Internet, blogs, journals and media

Activity 3.1   *Reflection*

Reflect on your last practice experience and consider the interactions and interventions you engaged in under the supervision of your mentor. For one of the patients/clients you cared for, identify the source of information that underpinned your actions. For example.

- Perhaps you were monitoring a patient's heart rate and respiration. How did you know whether the observations you recorded were within normal parameters? Where did the evidence for these limits come from?
- Perhaps you changed a patient's dressing? How did you know what dressing to use and when it should be changed next?
- Perhaps you were caring for a distressed patient or relative where you did not know what to say, but you instinctively placed your hand on their arm to convey your concern. What is the rationale for your action?

Once you have identified the type of evidence you used, consider where it sits within the hierarchy of evidence presented in Table 3.1.

Activity 3.1 continued

As this activity is based on your own practice, there is no outline answer at the end of the chapter.

It is important that nurses are able to provide a robust rationale for any source of evidence used to make decisions in practice, and to understand the nature of the source and any challenges that could be made against the integrity and validity of the evidence. This topic is explored in detail in two other books in this series: *Clinical Judgement and Decision Making in Nursing* and *Reflective Practice in Nursing*. In reality, it is not always possible to identify traditional evidence to support practice, so experience and intuition also have a role in decision making in areas that may be under-researched or complex, or in situations where decisions have to be made based on limited information. The next section will focus on current sources of evidence and identify issues relating to their reliability.

Sources of evidence

It is *essential* that you begin to learn to use some bibliographic databases, electronic journals and information gateways, in order to ensure that you can access material of good quality from a range of sources that will enable you to keep up to date with current practice. University libraries will normally offer workshops and online tutorials on how to use these professional sources of information. Make good use of these resources so that you continue to develop your searching skills over the course of your programme.

Intute (2010) offers an outline of the types of professional resources that you can use to support your assignments and professional practice, and these have been summarised in Table 3.2.

Table 3.2: Sources of information to support professional practice

Resource	Description and examples
Publications from key organisations	For example, Department of Health, World Health Organization, National Patient Safety Agency.
Electronic journals	These are becoming increasingly available, but many require subscription. Remember to find out what e-journals your university subscribes to in your subject area.
Bibliographic databases	The Cochrane Library and Pubmed offer free access to a range of evidence-based information.
	Other bibliographic databases such as CINAHL (Cumulative Index of Nursing and Allied Health Literature) and ASSIA (Applied Social Sciences Index and Abstracts) require a subscription and may be available through your university library.
Information gateways	These specialist websites are often organised under subject headings to provide access to specific web-based information. Intute is one example.

Table 3.2: continued

Resource	Description and examples
Library catalogues	These catalogues list all the print items owned by the library.
Professional organisations	For example, the NMC and the Royal College of Nursing (RCN) are two key nursing organisations that provide information to guide and direct nursing practice.
News and media	BBC News: Health and Guardian.co.uk: Health are two examples of sources of media-generated health information.
Web 2 technology	Blogs, wikis, podcasts and video sharing are becoming increasingly popular mechanisms for sharing information. However, these sites must be used with caution as the reliability of the information cannot always be established.

Source: Adapted from Wojciechowicz, L (2010), *Internet for Nursing*.

The nursing section of Intute has been developed by staff from the University of Nottingham and a visit is highly recommended as it can provide you with up-to-date information on key nursing sites. Intute also offers an excellent online tutorial site called the Virtual Training Suite. The tutorial designed for nurses can be accessed at **www.vts.intute.ac.uk/tutorial/nursing**. At this site it is possible to identify numerous links to recommended professional resources. Information is provided about each resource and you can collect the links to the sites relevant to your branch of nursing, which you can then email to yourself for future use. At the time of publication the future of Intute is uncertain and it is likely that changes may result in the site being maintained rather than updated; also, a charge may be introduced in the future if you wish to access the Virtual Training Suite. More details are available at **www.intute.ac.uk/blog/2010/04/12/intute-plans-for-thefuture-2010-and-beyond** or **http://intute.ac.uk/faq.html**.

Activity 3.2	*Research*

- As you work through the next section begin to collect the web addresses of sources you think have particular relevance to you.
- Collect a minimum of four links that you think will be useful to you in your studies and your practice.
- As you continue in your programme, collect more links (don't forget to add the web addresses included in your module bibliographies).
- Store these links safely as you will need to return to them in Chapter 4.

As this activity depends on your own studies, there is no outline answer at the end of the chapter.

The next section reviews sources that are relevant to nursing. It will begin with some that may already be familiar to you, but which have to be used with caution as the evidence they provide cannot always be authenticated.

Google Scholar™

If you are familiar with using Google™ search engine to find information, you may initially feel more comfortable beginning with this source. Like the generic Google search engine, Google Scholar™ scholarly texts search is a free online search tool that provides a search of scholarly literature from a range of sources such as theses, books and articles (Google Scholar, 2010).

Unlike Google, Google Scholar allows you to undertake a more precise search. Select the Advanced Scholar Search, as this not only allows you to be specific about the key words you use, it also allows you to search for specific authors or to limit your search by year of publication. Google Scholar also offers Advanced Scholar Search tips that help you make the most of this resource.

The disadvantage of using Google Scholar is that it will often only provide you with an abstract of the journal articles you find, and there is often a fee to access the full text. However, you may be able to access the full text article through your university library if your university subscribes to the journal in which the article is published. If this is not the case, your library may offer an interlibrary loan system for a limited number of requests, so you may still be able to access the full text through this process.

As with all sources of information, remember to record all the details required to correctly reference the literature you find. If any of the details are incomplete, for example author, publisher and place of publication, or if the journal/book title is missing, there may be a problem with demonstrating the reliability of the information you have found.

Wikipedia®

Wikipedia® is a very convenient source of information and may be one with which you are already familiar.

> Wikipedia is a . . . web-based, free-content encyclopedia project based . . . Wikipedia is written collaboratively by largely anonymous internet users who write without pay. Anyone with internet access can write and make changes to Wikipedia articles.
>
> (Wikipedia, 2010)

Activity 3.3	Critical thinking

Consider the description of Wikipedia offered in the direct quote above and identify the risks and benefits of using a source such as Wikipedia.

Compare your risks and benefits with the answers given at the end of the chapter.

Wikipedia is quick and easy to use, and as a first source of information it can be a useful introduction to a new topic. However, it is often difficult to identify the author/co-authors of material on this site and this therefore raises questions regarding reliability. Anyone can publish anonymously on this site, and as it is only weakly peer-reviewed, errors or malicious entries may remain accessible for a time before they are corrected or removed. Therefore, when using Wikipedia as a source as evidence, it is essential that you use additional, more reliable, sources of evidence to confirm the information you have found on Wikipedia.

Key organisations

Key organisations such as the Department of Health (DH) can be accessed through a generic search engine such as Google. Once on the DH site, it is reasonable to assume that the information it contains is reliable and based on credible evidence.

Department of Health

The Department of Health (**www.dh.gov.uk**) publishes many documents that contain standards, recommendations and guidance that are relevant to nursing and midwifery. The 'Health care' page provides links to all healthcare publications and to the National Service Frameworks (NSFs), which provide standards of care in a range of nursing and midwifery contexts such as children and maternity, coronary heart disease, mental health and diabetes.

Activity 3.4   *Research*

- Log on to the Department of Health at **www.dh.gov.uk**.
- Use the search facility to access an NSF relevant to your branch of nursing.
- Save the link to this site.

As this activity depends on your own field of practice, there is no outline answer at the end of the chapter.

This website also provides links to current news and updates as well as access to the NHS Evidence search portal, which *provides rapid access to information for everyone working in health and social care* (NHS Evidence, 2009).

National Institute for Health and Clinical Excellence

On its homepage, NICE (**www.nice.org.uk**) states that it is *an independent organisation responsible for providing national guidance on promoting good health and preventing ill health*. It provides the latest evidence-based guidelines, guidance implementation and quality initiatives and is a valuable source of clinical guidelines for nurses and other health professionals on a wide range of health topics.

Activity 3.5   *Research and reflection*

- Access the NICE website at **www.nice.org.uk**.
- Find the latest NICE guideline that relates to your field of practice, e.g. the management of type 2 diabetes, diabetes during pregnancy, fever management in children, or depression in adults.
- Consider how the practice you have experienced on your placement reflects the guidelines, and what challenges exist when implementing guidelines.

As this activity depends on your own field of practice, there is no outline answer at the end of the chapter.

NHS Institute for Innovation and Improvement

The NHS Institute for Innovation and Improvement (**www.institute.nhs.uk**) is part of the DH and is specifically focused on developing and disseminating new ways of working and new technology and on developing leadership. It provides practical frameworks for the improvement of the quality of care.

NHS National Patient Safety Agency

The NPSA (**www.npsa.nhs.uk**) has three sections and the National Reporting and Learning Services section provides information that can improve patient safety. The site has a range of resources, including teaching resources designed to improve risk management in practice.

Information gateways

Intute

At the time of publication, Intute (**www.intute.ac.uk**) is regularly updated, but from July 2011 it may just be maintained and not necessarily added to. However, details have been included here as currently it is a very useful resource.

Intute is a web-based resource that is organised by university subject specialists under subject headings. Each subject heading provides a brief description of each of the websites included. This site is an information gateway that includes only the sites most relevant to the subject headings, and is designed to make it easier to find subject-specific information. It is not a source of academic papers or journal articles.

Intute will not only identify government-based sites such as the DH, but will also identify sites that are service-user focused and that provide information for patients and carers. These are often useful sites where novice nurses can gain an insight into the ways in which illness and disease impact on patients' lives, before progressing on to more academic sources of information.

NHS libraries

NHS Evidence: Health Information Resources

As a student on a nursing or midwifery programme you can gain free access to NHS Evidence: Health Information Resources (formerly known as the National Library for Health). The National Library for Health transferred to NHS Evidence on 1 April 2009.

> NHS Evidence incorporates some of the key components from the National Library for Health, enhancing and providing the latest functionality. In addition, NHS Evidence is developing an accreditation process for sources of information to provide confidence for users of health and social care information.
>
> (NHS Evidence, 2010)

This excellent online resource is user-friendly and specifically designed to provide access to evidence-based reviews, the National Library of Guidelines, NICE guidelines, books, journals, healthcare databases and much more. You will need to register for an account to access some of these resources.

The site also has RSS feeds that allow information from this site to be brought direct to your computer without the need for searching. The use of RSS feeds will be explored in Chapter 5.

NHS Trust Libraries

When you are on placements you have the opportunity to access your NHS Trust's library. The Trust librarians can direct you to the free resources available to you as a nursing or midwifery student and inform you of any borrowing rights you may have.

University libraries

Unlike a public library, your university library will have its own website that will contain free resources purchased specifically for your programme. University websites will provide you with access to information from academic sources that cannot be accessed through your public library, Google or Google Scholar. It is important to take advantage of any library workshops relating to the use of the resources that are relevant to your nursing programme.

Your university library will contain a range of books and journals on the shelves, but this is only a small proportion of the information held. However, before embarking on a discussion of the electronic sources of information available to students, it is important to remember that your programme/module tutor will provide you with a bibliography listing the core text and recommended texts that they will expect you to read as part of your course. You should use the reference information in the bibliographies as the first stage in your search of the library catalogue.

Library catalogues

The library catalogue will provide access to the books, DVDs and printed journals held by your university library. University libraries aim to provide a number of copies of all the recommended books for your module or programme, but there will be a limited number, so you may like to consider buying some key textbooks. Ask your personal tutor, module leader or programme director for guidance on which books they recommend you purchase.

When searching the library catalogue it is easy to find what you want if you know the title or author of the book. However, if you do not have this information you need to remember that books contain a much wider range of information on a topic than a journal article, so the book title is likely to be broad rather than specific. For example, searching for pressure sores OR decubitus ulcers may be too precise search terms for the library catalogue. Searching for nursing care or tissue viability is more likely to provide an appropriate introduction to the topic within one of a textbook's chapters. You can also search the library catalogue by subject area, such as nursing care.

When searching the library catalogue it is important to make a note of the classmark of the book. The classmark is a series of numbers and/or letters that enables you to locate a book on the library shelves. If the book you want is already on loan you may find an alternative, suitable book on the shelves by looking at books with a similar classmark.

Libraries also contain records of all the journals or periodicals they subscribe to, and where they are located in the library. It is not advisable to search journals or periodicals by hand as an electronic search is a far more efficient use of time. However, if you have found a useful reference during a search on Google Scholar, you can use the library catalogue to search the list of journals held by the university to see if you can access a full-text hard copy for free. You can also search for journals by subject through the library catalogue. The catalogue will usually also hold details of video recordings, newspapers and large-print books.

E-books

The ability to access electronic books or online versions of printed books is an expanding area and is likely to increase dramatically over the coming years. Searching Google Books™

book search is a simple way to see if you can view a book or chapter online for free. Many universities also have access to e-books.

Bibliographic databases

Your university has to pay for access to bibliographic databases and you will be given a user name and password that will enable you to access these resources. This may be referred to as your library or ATHENS account.

A bibliographic database contains references to a vast range of published literature contained in journal articles, conference proceedings, reports, government publications and newspaper articles. Information is usually presented in the form of a reference and an abstract (or summary of the literature). Not all bibliographic databases provide access to the full text of all the information that is indexed. In these cases it may be necessary to record the reference and seek a full-text copy via your library's print or electronic holdings or through their interlibrary loan system.

If you have the name of a particular journal or subject area, you can search for it through your university library database, to see if the full text is available. Knowing the volume and issue number of the article you wish to find will greatly increase the likelihood of finding the article you need through e-journal searching.

When using bibliographic databases, it is important to use those that are the most relevant to your subject area. For nursing students CINAHL (Cumulative Index of Nursing and Allied Health Literature) and the British Nursing Index may the most useful, along with PsycINFO, which covers all aspects of psychology.

EBSCOhost's Electronic Journals Service (EJS) is one gateway to thousands of e-journals containing millions of articles from hundreds of different publishers, all at one website. This may be available to you via your university library website.

Medline includes literature relating to medicine, but also includes nursing and allied health literature. ASSIA is the Applied Social Sciences Index and Abstracts, a database that contains over 255,000 records dating back to 1987. This may be a useful source of information on a topic that has a social as well as a medical/nursing focus, for example domestic violence.

Choosing which source to search will be dependent on the topic. Use your university librarian to help you identify which sources are the most likely to contain the information you seek.

Activity 3.6   *Research*

Finding your way around the many resources your university library has to offer is *essential* if you wish to be successful in your studies. To make sure you are familiar with your university library resources:

- take a tour of the library (this may be a virtual tour or conducted by the librarians as part of your induction programme);
- find the 'book class' of the books related to your particular subject and find the section in the library where they are stored;
- find out where printed copies of nursing and midwifery journals are stored;
- sign up for any workshops run by the librarians that can help you become familiar with accessing the library catalogue, e-journals and bibliographic databases.

As this activity depends on the resources of your own university library, there is no outline answer at the end of the chapter.

National databases

The Cochrane Collaboration

The UK Cochrane Collaboration is one of 12 centres worldwide that facilitate and coordinate the publication of systematic reviews of randomised controlled trials. It also provides training for contributors. To search this site use the Cochrane Library webpage at **www.thecochranelibrary.com/view/o/index.html**.

Systematic reviews are seen as the most reliable source of evidence; however, such reviews will not exist for all areas where evidence is required.

Demographic information

The Office of National Statistics (ONS) is a source of demographic information related to England, Wales, Scotland and Northern Ireland:

> *[It] covers population and demographic information. It contains commentary on the latest findings, topical articles on relevant subjects such as one parent families, cohabitation, fertility differences, international demography, population estimates and projections for different groups. [It is] illustrated with colour charts and diagrams, regularly updated statistical tables and graphs, showing trends and the latest quarterly information on: conceptions, births, marriages, divorces, internal and international migration, population estimates and projections, etc.*
>
> (ONS, 2010)

Professional bodies and organisations

Nursing and Midwifery Council

The NMC is the statutory body set up to regulate the nursing and midwifery profession in the UK. The NMC website (**www.nmc-uk.org**) provides access to all the Council's standards, publications and consultations with which nurses and midwives have to comply.

The site also enables employers to check the registration status of their employees and to access information on current Fitness to Practise (FtP) hearings. The records of these hearings provide insight into the reasons why nurses may be removed from the nursing register and can make interesting reading.

Royal College of Nursing

The RCN was founded in 1916. It is a membership organisation made up mainly of registered nurses, but also includes student nurses and healthcare assistants. Its aim is to represent nurses and nursing, to promote excellence in practice and to influence healthcare policy (see the RCN website **www.rcn.org.uk/about us**). Services include free access to the extensive RCN library. Membership of this organisation also allows you access to its numerous publications and research. The RCN website also offers guidance on professional development that includes guides to using its library services.

News and the media

Newspapers and television

Newspapers and television often contain health information, but these sources need to be viewed with caution as they do not always present a complete or unbiased view of health topics. However, they do provide a source of information for the general public, so keeping up to date with the content of the health pages of newspapers, news programmes and documentaries can provide insight into patients' perspectives and expectations of healthcare provision.

These sources may provide a focus for exploring a topic, but they should not be used as the sole source of evidence to support or change practice. Rather, they should be viewed as a motivation for a more comprehensive and academic investigation.

Blogs

The personal knowledge and experiences of patients, clients and carers has been recognised by some as a valid source of information to inform clinical practice (Rycroft-Malone et al., 2004). Such information may be gathered in a variety of ways. Patient satisfaction surveys or audits of the patient experience provide quantitative data that can be utilised to improve the quality of service provision. Other sources of information may be much more difficult to utilise.

Blogs can provide a personal commentary on a particular topic such as politics or news, or be a form of personal online diary or journal. A blog is an individual record of an experience and provides a personal, subjective perspective on a topic. This must be remembered if you use the content of a blog as evidence to support your studies. For instance, you may come across the blog of a woman who has experienced breast cancer that would suggest practice could be improved for such patients. In this situation it is important to remember that this 'evidence' relates to the experience of one person and thus cannot be generalised to the experience of all patients with breast cancer. However, knowledge of a range of different patient experiences may enable you to be more sensitive to the individual responses and needs of patients with specific conditions, rather than adopting a 'one size fits all' approach.

Other sources of evidence

Experts

The *Concise Oxford Dictionary* describes an expert as *having special skill at a task or knowledge in a subject*. It is often a combination of knowledge, experience and skill that makes us regard others as experts in nursing, and during your time as a nursing student you will meet many different experts, including expert patients and expert carers. These experts will provide some of the evidence you will use to support your practice.

When you first begin your nursing career it may seem that everyone but you is an expert. In your placement your mentor will be the expert in nursing who will guide, supervise and assess your practice. Initially, it is likely that you will take such direction with little questioning, but as you progress you will need to become less dependent on direction from others and more reliant on your own developing expertise. Your knowledge of theoretical perspectives will increase as the course progresses, and it will become less acceptable to just ask your mentor for information as you will be increasingly expected to have investigated topics yourself. You will also be expected to be able to offer an evidence-based rationale for the care you deliver or when challenging the practice of others. This does not mean that you should not seek expert advice, but rather that you should actively seek to increase your own independent learning, so that you can engage in professional debate and make a positive contribution to enhancing patient care.

Professional colleagues can be an invaluable source of knowledge and information, but their views must not be accepted without criticism as knowledge in healthcare is continuously developing. It is everyone's professional responsibility to keep up to date with changes so that, when they become registered nurses they have a knowledge base sufficient to support their practice.

Anecdotal evidence

Words associated with the word 'anecdotal' include subjective, untrustworthy and undependable. Anecdotal evidence, therefore, would suggest that such evidence is not robust and is perhaps based more on hearsay, myths and rituals than hard evidence.

The contents of a blog could be called anecdotal, and yet the subjective account of a person's experience of an illness may provide powerful insight into the lived experiences of patients that nurses could use to enhance care. Narrative (storytelling) is increasingly being used as a means of exploring and identifying evidence, so it would seem that, in the future, there needs to be further clarification of the term 'anecdotal' to ensure that useful evidence is not lost at the same time as myth and ritual are eliminated.

Activity 3.7   *Reflection and research*

It is likely that this chapter has presented you with details of many sources of information that you are not familiar with. If this is the case, undertake the following exercise.

- Make a list of all the sources of information mentioned in this chapter.
- Tick those you are familiar with.
- Create a new list of four or five sources that you are unfamiliar with but that will be useful to you in your studies.
- Create a timetable of activities for the next month that will enable you to become familiar with these new resources. This may include attending library workshops and completing online tutorials.
- Use these sources to find information for your first assignment so that you become more confident in using them.
- In three months' time return to your list and pick one or two more resources to learn to use.

As this activity depends on your own field of study, there is no outline answer at the end of the chapter.

In this way you can steadily build the range of resources you can access easily. In addition, the more familiar you are with the resources the more likely you are to select the source most likely to provide you with the information you seek.

CHAPTER SUMMARY

This chapter has outlined how to develop a simple plan for finding information to inform your studies and your practice. It has covered the following aspects:

- the nature of 'evidence';
- sources of evidence.

Check how much you have learnt

Undertake the following short test to see how much you have learnt by completing this chapter. Answers are provided below.

1. Complete the following sentence.
.... and .... are traditionally seen as the 'best' evidence to support practice.
2. Name the four sources of evidence identified by Rycroft-Malone et al. (2004).
   i.
   ii.
   iii.
   iv.
3. Draw a line between each source in the left-hand column and the correct description on the right.

Source		Description
Source		*Description*
Intute		A bibliographic database that requires subscription from your university
CINAHL		Provides free access to reliable sources of evidence for NHS staff and students
Google Scholar		A free web-based encyclopaedia
NHS Evidence		An information gateway: a specialist website organised under subject headings
Wikipedia		A commercial search engine on which you can search scholarly literature, including theses, books, abstracts and articles

4. Complete the following sentence.
   News and media sources have to be used with caution because the information they contain may be .... or ....

Answers

1. *Systematic reviews* and *randomised controlled trials* are traditionally seen as the 'best' evidence to support practice.
2. The four sources of evidence identified by Rycroft-Malone et al. (2004) are:
   i.   research;
   ii. clinical experience;
   iii. patient experience;
   iv. information from the local context.

3. The sources and their correct descriptions are as follows.

Source	Description
Intute	An information gateway: a specialist website organised under subject headings
CINAHL	A bibliographic database that requires subscription from your university
Google Scholar	A commercial search engine on which you can search scholarly literature, including theses, books, abstracts and articles
NHS Evidence	Provides free access to reliable sources of evidence for NHS staff and students
Wikipedia	A free web-based encyclopaedia

4. News and media sources have to be used with caution because the information they contain may be *incomplete* or *biased*.

Activities: Outline answer

Activity 3.3: Critical thinking (page 45)

Benefits of Wikipedia	Risks of Wikipedia
Huge amounts of information available	Anyone can publish/amend content
Through collaboration enables information to accumulate from a number of sources	Information may be inaccurate
Free and easily accessed online	Contributors often anonymous so their authority cannot be verified.

Knowledge review

Having completed the chapter, how would you now rate your knowledge of the following topics?

	Good	Adequate	Poor
1. The range of evidence that can be used to support practice.			
2. The range of sources of evidence.			
3. The limitations of some sources of evidence.			

Where you're not confident in your knowledge of a topic, what will you do next?

Further reading

Rycroft-Malone, J (2008) Evidence-informed practice: from individual to context. *Journal of Nursing Management*, Special Issue 16(4): 404–8.

Rycroft-Malone, J, Seers, K, Titchen, A, Harvey, G, Kitson, A and McCormack, B (2004) An exploration of the factors that influence the implementation of evidence into practice. *Journal of Clinical Nursing*, 13: 913–24.

Useful websites

http://en.wikipedia.org/wiki/Main_Page Wikipedia.
http://news.bbc.co.uk/1/hi/health/default.stm BBC News: Health.
www.dh.gov.uk Department of Health.
www.google.com/support/scholar/bin/request.py Google Scholar Help.
www.guardian.co.uk/society/health *Guardian*: Health.
www.hse.ie/eng/about/Who/Population_Health/Health_Intelligence/Health_Intelligence_Work/Evidence_Based_Health_Care/Hierarchy_of_Evidence University of Sheffield: Hierarchy of evidence.
www.institute.nhs.uk NHS Institute for Innovation and Improvement.
www.intute.ac.uk Intute.
www.library.nhs.uk NHS Evidence: Health Information Resources.
www.nmc-uk.org Nursing and Midwifery Council.
www.npsa.nhs.uk NHS National Patient Safety Agency.
www.rcn.org.uk Royal College of Nursing.
www.statistics.gov.uk Office of National Statistics.

Chapter 4

Using information in your work

Draft NMC Standards for Pre-registration Nursing Education

This chapter will address the following draft competencies:

Domain: Professional values

9. All nurses must recognise the limits of their own competence and knowledge. They must reflect on their own practice and seek advice from, or refer to, other professionals where necessary.
10. All nurses must practise independently, within their own limitations, and apply relevant theory and research to their practice. They must also recognise how different research methods are used to increase knowledge in nursing.

Domain: Nursing practice and decision making

6. All nurses must use a range of information and data to improve the health of individuals and populations, and support decision making. They must help people and their carers make choices about their health care needs.
9. All nurses must use up-to-date knowledge to decide the best way to deliver safe, evidence-based care across all ages.

Domain: Leadership, management and team working

10. All nurses must draw on a range of resources to evaluate and audit care, and then use this information to contribute to improving people's experience and outcomes of care and the shaping of future services.

Draft Essential Skills Clusters

This chapter will address the following draft ESCs:

Cluster: Organisational aspects of care

10. People can trust the newly registered graduate nurse to deliver nursing interventions and evaluate their effectiveness against the agreed assessment and care plan.

By the second progression point:

iv. Actively seeks to extend knowledge and skills using a variety of methods in order to enhance care delivery.

15. People can trust the newly registered graduate nurse to safely delegate to others and to respond appropriately when a task is delegated to them.

By entry to the register:

v. Recognises and addresses deficits in knowledge and skill in self and others and takes appropriate action.

Chapter aims

After reading this chapter, you will be able to:

- understand the importance of reading and note taking;
- paraphrase information and reference correctly in order to avoid plagiarism in your academic work;
- use evidence effectively to support your academic work and in practice.

Introduction

Having learnt how to find a range of reliable information sources relating to a specific topic, the next stage is to ensure that you use them effectively in your academic work. This chapter will enable you to understand how, by effective reading, note taking, critical thinking, practice experiences and reflection, you can make maximum use of the information available to inform your practice and your assignments.

The chapter will begin with a discussion on the importance of reading. This section also highlights the importance of graduate skills in academic work, and how good time management and organisational skills can enhance academic achievement and knowledge for practice.

Why is reading so important?

Reading is an important preparatory stage to examinations and writing assignments because it is the basis on which your success in academic studies is founded. Reading must begin before you start to plan your assignments, and this is why effective searching skills will help you find material efficiently and leave you time to read.

Personal experience as a university lecturer suggests that some students write their assignments based on limited knowledge and then try to find literature that will support their views. This approach to academic work will lead to superficial and subjective assignments that may result in academic failure or mediocre work that reflects limited knowledge and understanding of the topic.

Reading relevant literature allows you to develop depth in your initial understanding of a topic, and enables you to begin to consider any conflicting or counter arguments that emerge from the information you have accessed. This may direct you to other literature that will add to the depth and breadth of your knowledge of a subject, and enhance your ability to debate and evaluate the information on the topic.

Reading widely increases the need to be organised so that you can easily find the sections of the literature you wish to use in your assignment. Using a highlighter pen to mark relevant text in articles is one method of doing this, but you still have to scan all the highlighted text in the article before you find the information you need. Although this approach can be useful when reading articles, it is not one that you can use for other sources, such as books.

An alternative way to capture the information you need is to make notes as you read, translating the text you are reading into your own words. In this way you can avoid plagiarising others' work, and you can note any direct quotes that are of use to you. A scenario of how these notes could be developed is provided below.

Scenario: Note taking

You have been set the task of writing an essay on the nature of nursing.

Using lined paper with a left-hand margin, you can create notes on the literature that you need to support your essay, as shown below.

Reference:	Smith, H (2010) What is nursing? Nursing in UK 1(1): 33–42
page 33	Makes reference to Henderson's definition of nursing
	'to assist the individual, sick or well, in the performance of those activities contributing to health or its recovery (or to peaceful death) that he would perform unaided if he had the necessary strength, will, or knowledge. And to do this in such a way as to help him gain independence as rapidly as possible . . . This aspect of her work, this part of her function, she initiates and controls; of this she is master.'
	Cited from Henderson, V (1960) Basic principles of nursing care. London: ICN.
	This definition does not make any reference to working as part of a team but I think it does suggest that nurses are about enabling people to regain their health or manage their illness/disability, which seems relevant today.
	**Need to find other definitions and compare.
p35	Makes reference to Carper (1978), who suggested that nurses use a combination of knowledge – aesthetic, empirical, personal and ethical in order to deliver care. This does not necessarily tell you what nursing is, but is more about where nurses get their knowledge to underpin their practice.
p39	Makes reference to a report called 'The Prime Minister's Commission on the Future of Nursing and Midwifery in England'. *I need to access this report and see how the political view of nursing in the future differs from Henderson's vision. This might create some interesting discussion points.
p42	The article drifts into rather vague discussion and does not come to any specific conclusions, other than suggesting that nursing is a complex profession and one that continues to evolve over time in response to the needs of the population.

This approach to note keeping will enable you to quickly and easily review the key points in the information you have read. Recording the details of the reference at the top of the page means you will always have this available for your reference list. By noting the page numbers in your margin you can easily return to the original source of the notes to clarify what you have written. It also means that, when you come to write your essay, you simply have your notes to refer to rather than a pile of books and articles.

This is not the only approach to note taking, but whatever method you use to identify the key elements of the information you read, it needs to be one that works for you and enables you to retrieve information quickly to support your work once you start to write.

Once you have read and developed an understanding of the topic, you are then at the point where you can plan your assignment.

Paraphrasing and referencing

When using the information you have found in your academic work, you need to ensure that you acknowledge the source. Using direct quotes from any source of information must be accompanied by a reference to the author that includes the page number. For example, the direct quote cited in the above scenario would be included in your essay in the following format:

> to assist the individual, sick or well, in the performance of those activities contributing to health or its recovery (or to peaceful death) that he would perform unaided if he had the necessary strength, will, or knowledge. And to do this in such a way as to help him gain independence as rapidly as possible . . . This aspect of her work, this part of her function, she initiates and controls; of this she is master.
>
> Henderson (1960, cited in Smith, 2010, p33)

This direct quote is a secondary reference (that is, taken from Smith's book not the original work by Henderson). Wherever possible, try to access the primary source of information in order to have a more comprehensive understanding of the original concepts.

Note that the direct quote is indented from the margins and the page number of the source is included. Definitions such as this are often used as direct quotes, but are of little value if you do not comment on them to demonstrate your understanding. For example, you could write 'This definition suggests that nursing is . . .'

Paraphrasing is summarising the information you have read into your own words. If we take the Henderson quote above, you could paraphrase this as follows:

> Henderson's definition of nursing (1960, cited in Smith, 2010) still appears to have relevance to nursing today, as it suggests that nursing is concerned with enabling individuals to gain independence in their healthcare needs through the support and guidance of the nurse.

Paraphrasing allows you to demonstrate what you have understood from reading, and critically evaluating a range of information and applying this to a specific situation. It demonstrates higher-level thinking and also promotes a more discursive style of academic writing.

How much do you need to read?

Students often ask how much they need to read and therefore how many references they need for their essays. This is a difficult question to answer as it will be different depending on the essay topic. For instance, if you are completing a research critique you may only use two or three references to current research textbooks, one or two references to critiquing frameworks and reference to the research study you are critiquing. For other health topics, such as obesity, there would be much more literature available that would include research studies on obesity, health promotion, nutrition and government policy. As a consequence, the marker would expect you to use a wider range of literature on the topic of obesity than necessarily expected for a research critique.

However, as a general rule, for a first-year piece of work you should plan to read a *minimum* of four relevant sources of information for every 1,000 words of an essay. This means that a 3,000-word essay should use a least 12 different sources of information to support the work. This should rise to six to eight sources per 1,000 words by the time you are in year three of your programme. However, all universities differ, so it is important that you seek guidance from the module/programme leader and assignment guidelines so that you are confident you have accessed sufficient information to support each assignment.

Can you read too much?

It could be seen as unhelpful to discourage you from reading widely, but occasionally a student becomes so absorbed in a topic and reads so widely that he or she does not leave enough time to absorb and process all the information into a coherent essay. This will result in an essay grade that does not accurately reflect the amount of student effort. As with searching for information, it is important to set yourself a time limit for reading. You will need to identify a point at which you will stop reading and begin to plan and write your essay. Once you have a first draft of an essay completed, you could then make use of any time available to extend your reading and add further depth to your discussion.

Getting side-tracked

When reading for an assignment, you may come across information you find fascinating but that is only distantly related to the focus of your essay. The temptation is to try to change the focus of the essay to allow you to include this interesting information. You need to be wary of this, as it may well mean that you write a very interesting and well-researched essay, but fail the assignment because it does not fully address the assignment task.

Make reading professional information a regular feature of each week

Try to establish the habit of regular reading of professional journals relevant to your particular branch of nursing. This will not only enable you to keep up to date with current developments in your field, but will develop a broad-based professional knowledge that will complement the reading you are required to complete for your assignments. It is a habit that will then be well established once you qualify, and will support your continuing professional development as a registered practitioner.

- Look in your diary for the next month and identify time slots of between 40 and 60 minutes where you may have time for reading. For example, you may make regular bus or train trips, or have a dentist's or doctor's appointment where waiting to be seen is a possibility.
- Reflect on your normal daily routine and identify other 40- to 60-minute slots where you often have a little time to spare, e.g. first thing in the morning; between getting home and going to the gym/preparing an evening meal; or waiting to pick up your child from school or a club.
- Now draw up a daily timetable for the next month, identifying all the possible reading time slots you could use.
- Prepare a folder containing a notebook and reading material that you keep with you, so that you can make use of any unexpected delays that can be filled with reading.
- Over the next month try using the time slots you have identified for reading.
- Reflect on your experience and identify the times you consider have been the most productive reading times.
- Use this reduced number of time slots to plan your reading for the next month.

As this activity depends on your personal circumstances, there is no outline answer at the end of the chapter.

By planning in this way, reading is a steady process that allows you time to assimilate one lot of information before moving on to the next. It will allow you time to identify and explore any contradictions in the information you have accessed and begin to develop critical insight into the topic. As you become more informed by your reading, you will be able to ask relevant questions of your module teacher and participate more confidently in classroom debate.

Using the information in your academic work

Having found and read the information, you need to maximise your effort by using it effectively to support your academic work. This will be explored in three sections: demonstrating what you know, using information to develop analysis and evaluation, and application of theory to practice.

Demonstrating what you know

Presenting a sound level of knowledge and understanding is essential to pass any assignment, but the first task is to be confident that you understand what knowledge you need to demonstrate for each assignment. This can be achieved by carefully reading the assignment guidelines and the programme/module learning outcomes, which will also be a source of key words for your search for information. All assignments are designed to measure the programme/module learning outcomes.

Activity 4.2   Critical thinking

- Access one of your module/programme handbooks and find the description of the intended learning outcomes. Read them and think about what evidence you will need to produce in your assignment to demonstrate that you have achieved these learning outcomes.
- Now turn to the section that describes the assessment for the module/programme. You should be able to see a clear link between the learning outcomes and the module/programme assignment.

Considering the learning outcomes and assignment guidelines should ensure that you stay focused on the assignment task.

As this activity depends on your own module/programme, there is no outline answer at the end of the chapter.

Demonstrating what you know about a topic forms the foundation on which analysis and critical evaluation are built. It tends to be descriptive. However, there are two types of descriptive writing: one type tells a story (anecdotal) and gains little in terms of marks, while the other type demonstrates knowledge, understanding and the use of literature, and contributes to the mark secured for an assignment.

Activity 4.3   Critical thinking

Read the example below and decide what type of descriptive writing it is.

Obesity is an enormous problem facing the UK at the moment. Increasing numbers of children and adults are being identified as being obese, which puts them at risk of developing serious health problems in the future.

Read on for an answer to this activity.

This is anecdotal writing, because it is written as personal opinion and is not supported by evidence from the literature. Below is another example of descriptive writing on the topic of obesity that is not anecdotal but academic, and that uses information from a range of sources.

Scenario: Descriptive writing

Obesity is described as an excess of body fat and is usually measured using the Body Mass Index (BMI) (NHS Information Centre, 2010). A BMI is calculated by dividing a person's weight measurement (in kilograms) by the square of their height (in metres). Individuals with a BMI over 30 are considered obese and a waist circumference in excess of 102 cm for men and 88 cm for women is also an indicator of obesity at a level likely to impact on health (NICE, 2006).

The number of obese people in the UK has increased from 13 per cent in 1993 to 24 per cent in 2008 for men, and from 16 per cent to 25 per cent for women (Health

Scenario continued

Survey for England, 2008). By 2012 it is predicted that 32.1 per cent of men and 31 per cent of women will be obese (Zaninotto, 2009).

Obesity has been described as:

a major public health problem due to its association with serious chronic diseases such as type 2 diabetes, hypertension (high blood pressure), and hyperlipidaemia (high levels of fats in the blood that can lead to narrowing and blockages of blood vessels), which are major risk factors for cardiovascular disease and cardiovascular related mortality.

(NHS Information Centre, 2010, p49)

It is also associated with cancer, disability and reduced quality of life, and can lead to premature death.

Now you have read the two examples above, complete Activity 4.4.

Activity 4.4   *Critical thinking*

Compare the two examples of descriptive writing above and identify why the second example makes better use of the information accessed than the first.

An outline answer to this activity is given at the end of the chapter.

These examples are intended to illustrate how you can demonstrate that you have accessed a range of information to support your work and also show a sound knowledge of the topic. The next stage is to move your work from a description of the information you have discovered to a critical analysis of the topic. This is explored in depth in another book in this series, *Critical Thinking and Writing for Nursing Students*. However, one simple example is included below.

Developing analysis in your work

Developing analysis in your work requires you to have accessed and read sufficient information to identify a range of perspectives on the topic for consideration. You can then begin to analyse each element and develop a critical discussion on the topic. Using the scenario on descriptive writing above, analysis could be introduced by adding the following.

Scenario: Introducing analysis

This data suggests that not only does obesity place individuals at greater risk of disease and premature death, but that the number at risk is rising at an approximate rate of 4 per cent annually. Any increase in illness or disease resulting from obesity will place increased demand on the resources of the National Health Service that could be avoided. This goes some way towards explaining the current policy drivers aimed at reducing rates of obesity (DH, 2010, 2006; NICE, 2006).

The scenario draws together the information given in the previous scenario, and provides an interpretation that demonstrates understanding of the information and the ability to draw conclusions (analyse) relating to its significance.

The example of analysis is the writer's interpretation of the literature he or she has read. There are some useful phrases, given in Table 4.1, that you can use to encourage you to think and write critically.

Table 4.1: Thinking and writing critically

Thinking critically	Writing critically
So why is this important?	This would seem to suggest that . . .
What are the implications of this information?	The implications of this appear to be . . .
Is this the only perspective?	This view has been challenged by Smith (2010), who implies that . . .
Does this fit with my experience in practice?	This may be difficult to implement in practice because . . .

You will note that the statements in the critical writing column are conditional, using words such as *seem to, appear to, could* and *may be*. This is important because you are expressing your own interpretation and judgement, and not expressing definitive facts.

When you review the first draft of your work, ask yourself the questions in the critical thinking column at the end of each of the paragraphs of your essay and check that you have made a critical or evaluative written statement in each. Revising your work in this way will enable you to ensure that you embed analysis throughout your essay and make explicit the depth of the knowledge and understanding you have gained through your reading and from your practice experiences.

Application of theory to practice

Making links between theory and practice is not always easy. However, making links between theoretical perspectives or research evidence and practice is another way of demonstrating knowledge and understanding, and the ability to analyse and synthesise information.

Continuing with the example of obesity, mental health nursing students may wish to focus on the psychological impact obesity can have on aspects of mental health, such as self-esteem, as well as on conditions such as depression. Using examples from mental health practice may challenge solutions purely focused on the physical health problems associated with obesity, and expose the complexity of such health issues.

Adult and child nursing students working in the acute setting may face a different challenge in practice, as they will need to move away from a medical model of treatment and cure to one where opportunistic health promotion will be an expectation. Adults and children admitted to acute units will need to have their BMIs calculated and health advice given to those who fall into the overweight or obese categories even if their weight is not the reason for admission. However, there is a need to deliver these messages sensitively and at a time when the patient/carer is likely to be receptive to health promotion messages. This may involve sharing patient information with other agencies that are better placed to provide long-term advice and support, for example a practice nurse (or a health visitor/school nurse in the case of a child).

Using information to inform your practice

Evidence-based practice in nursing is explored in another book in this series, so this section will explore how you can use practice information to maximise your learning from practice placements.

The NMC (2010) stipulates that all nursing students must complete a minimum of 2,300 hours in practice so that students can gain competence in a range of skills needed to deliver safe and effective care. However, placements are for much more than just learning clinical skills. They are concerned with facilitating the development of professional behaviours, team working and the promotion of good-quality care that is underpinned by reliable evidence. This section will consider how you can use information before, during and after placements to enhance your learning.

Before your placements

Your university will prepare you for your placements, but it is also your responsibility as a student to access relevant information in the weeks preceding your placements. This information is often provided online. Your placement administrator/coordinator will provide information regarding placement location and contact details.

Prior to any placement there is key information you need to find out, including:

- the location of the placement, and its telephone number and postcode;
- any particular access requirements (e.g. if you need a door code to gain access);
- parking or public transport information;
- the URL of any web-based information;
- uniform requirements (e.g. if you are required to wear uniform or smart/casual clothing);
- shift patterns and your own off-duty hours;
- the name of your mentor and where to meet on the first day.

Once you have accessed this information you need to plan your learning. However, before you begin to plan you need to know enough about the placement to be able to anticipate what learning opportunities might be available that you can develop into a learning contract. Some of these will have been made clear during your placement preparation at the university; however, each placement will also have some specific learning opportunities linked to the nature of the placement. For example, you may be placed on a nurse-led minor injuries unit as part of an acute service placement. Here you could expect to learn about nursing assessment and measuring vital signs; however, in addition there would be opportunities to learn about triage and taking a patient history, as well as to gain clinical skills such as injection techniques, applying wound dressings and observing suturing.

Such information about the nature of a placement can then be used to develop a draft learning contract for discussion with your mentor on your first day. Do not forget to include areas for development identified in previous placements; for example, a previous mentor may have identified that you need to build your confidence in providing discharge advice for patients. You will need to seek opportunities to provide discharge advice on your next placement.

Using information in this way to prepare for your placement will enable your mentor to plan your learning from your first day and to make sure that your learning outcomes are realistic in terms of the placement, your level of competence and the opportunities available. It will also demonstrate your ability to take responsibility for your own learning.

In Chapter 1 you used a SWOT analysis and SMART objectives to create a personal development plan. You can use the same principles to develop your learning contract for each practice placement experience. Within this contract you will include the specific learning outcomes for the placement identified in your preparation, plus any personal outcomes identified during previous placements.

Activity 4.5   *Evidence-based practice and reflection*

Consider the objectives identified in the left-hand column below. Complete the other columns.

Learning Contract: Surgical Ward
20 September 2010

Specific objectives	How will I know when it is achieved?	What resources will I need?	When will this be achieved by?
1. Safely prepare patients for surgery			
2. Understand the evidence base of pre- and post-operative care			
3. Effectively monitor patients' vital signs during pre- and post-operative recovery			
4. Recognise early signs of deterioration			
5. Provide appropriate discharge information for uncomplicated surgical cases			

Compare your learning contract with that given at the end of the chapter.

Accessing information on placement

On the first day of your placement you should be offered an orientation so that you are aware of the layout of the area, fire exits, emergency call systems, the location of emergency equipment and emergency procedures. This will allow you to respond appropriately in an emergency situation.

Other important information to access is the formal policies and procedures of the organisation in which you are placed. These will relate to a wide range of issues, such as infection control procedures, lone working policies and referral processes. Accessing and reading such policies enables you to work to the standards expected of that organisation. Use your mentor to guide you to those policies you need to familiarise yourself with first, and use your own initiative to identify policies that relate to patients in your care.

In clinical practice the patients are an excellent learning resource. Ask permission to read their notes and use the information you gain to seek further guidance from sources such as NICE and NHS Evidence in order to find information regarding best practice. Consider the medication your patient is receiving; do you understand how it works and any contraindications or adverse effects associated with its use? Was there a clear rationale for the nursing care plan supported with evidence?

Talk to your patients and listen to their experience and perception of illness and treatments, and reflect on what they have told you. However, it is very important to note that patient information is confidential and their information can only be shared on a need-to-know basis with those professionals engaged in their care. Patients' notes should not be photocopied or used in any way that could allow confidential information to be shared without their permission.

On your placements you will have access to your mentor, other experienced nurses and other expert professionals, all of whom will have information that you can use to enhance and examine your practice. To access this knowledge you will need to formulate appropriate questions and have the confidence to ask them.

You must also be willing to accept both positive and negative feedback on your performance from patients, your mentor and other professionals, and take action to address any areas that need improvement and value those aspects of your practice where your performance is good.

During your placement it is important to keep a record of your experience as well as your thoughts and feelings, so that you can use it to reflect on your placement once it has been completed. This record could take the form of a journal or diary of events.

Reflection on practice experience

Practice experience is a rich source of information to reflect on in order to learn from your placements. Making explicit your practice learning can enable you to enhance your practice and add depth to analysis within assignments by demonstrating your ability to apply theory to practice.

Models of reflection are designed to guide students and practitioners through this process and typically include:

- a description of the experience and associated feelings;
- an evaluation of the experience;
- an analysis of the experience;
- an action plan for future learning/behaviour.

The use of a journal to record details of experiences and feelings is promoted as an important feature of the description element of the process of reflection. Another book in this series, *Reflective Practice in Nursing*, offers further information on the reflection process.

When an assignment requires you to reflect on an incident in practice, the process is slightly different as it would not be appropriate to include your entire reflective log in an assignment. When writing a reflective essay the descriptive element (your log entries) needs to be succinct and focused on a key issue or issues as outlined below.

Concept summary: Writing reflective essays

Description	The description of the experience needs to be brief but sufficient to set the experience within a context.
Evaluation	This section should identify the good and bad aspects of the experience and identify the key issues to be explored.
Analysis	This will be the largest section of any reflective assignment. It will explore relevant literature, alternative perspectives and changes in your own attitudes and values that may result from this process.
Action plan	In this final section you will need to identify what you have learnt from reflecting on this experience and how this will impact on your future practice. This section can provide the conclusion to your essay.

The example below is a reflective essay from a student who was working on a neonatal care unit.

Scenario: Worked example of a reflective essay

Description	'The first stage of any reflection on practice is a description of the experience (Gibbs, 1998). The experience took place on a regional neonatal intensive care unit (NICU). I was working with my mentor (a junior staff nurse) in the NICU when a team of doctors arrived to examine the neonates in our care. As the consultant moved from one neonate to the next I realised that he had not washed his hands. I was aware that I needed to intervene in order to safeguard my patients, but hesitated as the doctor was a consultant and he had a group of other doctors and medical students with him. At this moment my mentor called the consultant to one side and reminded him that he needed to wash his hands. He thanked my mentor for reminding him, washed his hands and proceeded to the next patient.'
Evaluation	'When evaluating this incident it raised several issues for me, both good and bad. The positive aspect was the behaviour of my mentor. She was assertive, confident and yet respectful of the position and status of the consultant. The response of the consultant was also positive, in respecting the role the staff nurse played in ensuring that all staff followed infection control procedures.
	The negative aspects are the belief that, if my mentor had not been there, I do not think I would have challenged the consultant

---

Scenario continued

	and would have exposed my patients to unnecessary risk of harm. It also highlighted my perception of medical staff. I was surprised when the consultant thanked my mentor for intervening, as I expected him to be rude or aggressive in his response.'
Analysis	'Having completed the evaluation section, the next stage of reflection is analysis. In order for me to learn from this incident, the literature related to the concepts of accountability, assertive communication, perception, stereotyping and role modelling will be analysed in order to make sense of the learning that has occurred and how this will impact on my future behaviour. Accountability . . .'
Action plan	'In conclusion, exploring this incident has enabled me to recognise areas of weakness that I need to improve and to acknowledge the powerful influence of an excellent mentor and role model. These aspects will then be developed into an action plan as the final stage of the reflection process. I have learnt . . . In the future I will . . .'

Signposting

If using a model of reflection to structure analysis of an aspect of your reflective log, it is important not only to make reference to a specific model of reflection, but also to signpost your work. Signposting indicates where in the assignment you are using the model.

Activity 4.6 *Critical thinking*

Identify where signposting has been used in the above scenario.

Check your answers with those provided at the end of the chapter.

Clinical supervision

Mental health has an established tradition of using clinical supervision to enhance the process of reflection. Clinical supervision involves another professional who is trained to facilitate a discussion of casework or professional issues in order to assist the practitioner to reflect and learn from experience and improve their practice.

C H A P T E R   S U M M A R Y

This chapter has enabled you to understand how, by effective reading, note taking, critical thinking, practice experiences and reflection, you can make maximum use of the information available to inform your practice and your assignments.

Check how much you have learnt

Undertake the following short test to see how much you have learnt by completing this chapter. Answers are provided below.

1. List three reasons why reading is an essential preparation for assignment writing.
    i.
    ii.
    iii.
2. Which of the following statements is correct?
    i.   Read at least two sources of information per 1,000 words.
    ii. Read at least 12 sources of information per 3,000 words for an assignment in year 1.
    iii. Read a minimum of 18 sources of information per 300-word assignment in year 3.
    iv. Make sure every paragraph has at least one reference.
3. List three ways in which you can ensure that you understand what knowledge you need to develop for your assignments.
    i.
    ii.
    iii.
4. When you review the draft of your assignment, what questions should you ask yourself in order to check that you have developed analysis in your work?
    i.
    ii.
    iii.
    iv.
5. Draw a line between each element of the reflection process and its correct statement.

Element		Statement
Description		In this final section you will need to identify what you have learnt from reflecting on this experience and how this will impact on your future practice. This section can provide the conclusion to your essay.
Evaluation		This will be the largest section of any reflective assignment. It will explore relevant literature, alternative perspectives and changes in your own attitudes and values that may result from this process.
Analysis		The description of the experience needs to be brief but sufficient to set the experience within a context.
Action plan		This section should identify the good and bad aspects of the experience and identify the key issues to be explored.

Answers

1. Three reasons why reading is an essential preparation for assignment writing are:
   i. it forms the basis of academic success;
   ii. it allows the development of knowledge and understanding;
   iii. it promotes the consideration of different perspectives on a topic.
2. The following statement is correct:
   ii. Read at least 12 sources of information per 3,000 words for an assignment in year 1.
3. Three ways in which you can ensure that you understand what knowledge you need to develop for your assignments are:
   i. by accessing and reading literature from the module bibliography and starting to construct a list of key words;
   ii. by carefully reading the assignment title and guidelines and adding to your list of key words;
   iii. by reading the learning outcomes and identifying any additional key words for your search for information.
4. When you review the draft of your assignment, the questions you should ask yourself to check that you have developed analysis in your work are as follows.
   i. So why is this important?
   ii. What are the implications of this information?
   iii. Is this the only perspective?
   iv. Does this fit with my experience in practice?
5. The elements of the reflection process and their correct statements are as follows.

Element	Statement
Description	The description of the experience needs to be brief but sufficient to set the experience within a context.
Evaluation	This section should identify the good and bad aspects of the experience and identify the key issues to be explored
Analysis	This will be the largest section of any reflective assignment. It will explore relevant literature, alternative perspectives and changes in your own attitudes and values that may result from this process.
Action plan	In this final section you will need to identify what you have learnt from reflecting on this experience and how this will impact on your future practice. This section can provide the conclusion to your essay.

Activities: brief outline answers

Activity 4.4: Critical thinking (page 63)

The second example of descriptive writing will gain marks for the following reasons.

- It demonstrates depth of knowledge and understanding of the subject area.
- There is evidence of wide reading from a range of current and relevant sources of information.
- All statements are supported by a reference to a current published source.
- It is written in a clear and concise manner.
- It is correctly referenced.

Activity 4.5: Reflection (page 66)

A learning contract for a surgical placement could look like this.

Learning Contract: Surgical Ward
20 September 2010

Specific objectives	How will I know when it is achieved?	What resources will I need?	When will this be achieved by?
1. Safely prepare patients for surgery	Can effectively prepare booked patients for theatre with minimum direction from my mentor	• Opportunity to observe my mentor preparing patients for theatre • Opportunities to follow a surgical patient through from admission to discharge • Opportunity to admit and prepare a patient for theatre and receive feedback on my performance	• Formative assessment • Summative assessment
2. Understand the evidence base of pre- and post-operative care	Can provide an evidence based rationale for care provided for surgical patients	• Access to research related to pre- and post-operative care and discuss with mentor	• Summative assessment
3. Effectively monitor patients' vital signs during pre- and post-operative recovery	Can accurately record vital signs and recognise any deviation from normal	• Mentor will monitor my performance and provide feedback	• Formative assessment

4. Recognise early signs of deterioration	Use observation skills and EWS to ensure any deterioration in the patient is detected early	• Seek opportunities to participate in the care of a patient whose condition is unstable	• Summative assessment
5. Provide appropriate discharge information for uncomplicated surgical cases	When feedback from mentor and patient suggests all relevant information provided	• Opportunities to provide discharge information under supervision of my mentor	• Formative assessment

Activity 4.6: Critical thinking (page 69)

The phrases in the scenario on pages 68–9 below that are signposting the various elements of the reflection process are as follows.

- **Description**: 'The first stage of any reflection on practice is a description of the experience.'
- **Evaluation**: 'When evaluating this incident . . .'
- **Analysis**: '. . . the next stage of reflection is analysis.'
- **Action plan**: 'These will then be developed into an action plan as the final stage of the reflection process.'

Knowledge review

Having completed the chapter, how would you now rate your knowledge of the following topics?

	Good	Adequate	Poor
1. The importance of reading.			
2. How to demonstrate your knowledge and understanding in essays.			
3. How to use the information you have found.			
4. Using information in your assignments.			
5. Using information from your practice.			

Where you're not confident in your knowledge of a topic, what will you do next?

Further reading

Fowler, J (2006) The organization of clinical supervision within the nursing profession: a review of the literature. *Journal of Advanced Nursing*, 23(3): 471–8.

Howatson-Jones, L (2010) *Reflective Practice in Nursing.* Exeter: Learning Matters.

Price, R and Harrington, A (2010) *Critical Thinking and Writing for Nursing Students.* Exeter: Learning Matters.

Useful websites

www.connectingforhealth.nhs.uk/systemsandservices/infogov/caldicott Caldicott Guardians (patient confidentiality).

www.nmc-uk.org/Nurses-and-midwives/Advice-by-topic/A/Advice/Confidentiality NMC advice on confidentiality.

Chapter 5
Managing electronic information

Draft NMC Standards for Pre-registration Nursing Education

This chapter will address the following draft competencies:

Domain: Professional values

8. All nurses must be responsible and accountable for keeping their own knowledge and skills up-to-date through continuing professional development and life-long learning. They must use evaluation, supervision and appraisal to improve their performance and enhance the safety and quality of care and service delivery.

Domain: Communication and interpersonal skills

2. All nurses must use a range of communication skills and technologies to support person-centred care and enhance the quality and safety of healthcare. They must make sure that people receive all the information they need about their care in a language and manner that is right for them, and that allows them to make informed choices and consent to treatment.

Domain: Leadership, management and team working

5. All nurses must continue their professional development, supporting the professional and personal development of others, demonstrating leadership, reflective practice, supervision, quality improvement and teaching skills.

Draft Essential Skills Clusters

This chapter will address the following draft ESCs:

Cluster: Organisational aspects of care

14. People can trust the newly registered graduate nurse to be autonomous and confident as a member of the multi-disciplinary or multi-agency team and to inspire confidence in others.

By the second progression point:

v. Communicates with colleagues verbally, face-to-face and by telephone, and in writing and electronically in a way that the meaning is clear, and checks that the communication has been fully understood.

Chapter aims

After reading this chapter, you will be able to:

- demonstrate knowledge of a range of effective systems that facilitate the management of electronic/digital information that will enable you to keep up to date with evidence in your field of practice.

Please note that you will find it useful to be logged on to the internet while working your way through this chapter.

Introduction

Chapter 2 encouraged the development of your digital literacy skills and Chapter 3 offered guidance on how to access a range of electronic sources of information. Now, this chapter will focus on exploring the various methods that exist to help you access and store electronic/digital information efficiently. It is also designed to help you develop ways of facilitating information to come to you.

The chapter is sequenced in order of complexity with the simplest approaches to managing information provided first and the more complex approaches later.

Storing web addresses

If you are familiar with using Favorites (note the US spelling) in Microsoft Internet Explorer® or Bookmarks in other browsers such as Google Chrome™ browser or Mozilla Firefox, skip this section and move on to the section on Delicious.

When searching for information on the web it can be very frustrating when you move away from a useful website and then are unable to find it again. If you have experienced this problem, you will appreciate how useful it is to have a simple system that will allow you to store the URL details of these websites on your computer. As all websites have an address called a URL (discussed on page 30) they can be saved and stored in a variety of ways, including using Favorites, bookmarks and facilities such as Delicious. These enable you to create folders in which you can organise the URLs, thus making retrieval straightforward.

Favorites and Bookmarks

The screenshot in Figure 5.1 illustrates how Favorites can be accessed from Microsoft Internet Explorer. Clicking on Favorites provides access to a drop-down menu that allows you to save the URL and give the site a title that will enable you to file and easily retrieve it in the future. It is possible to change the title that it is stored under in your Favorites by right-clicking the Favorite, selecting Rename, and then overtyping the original title.

To add a Favorite in Internet Explorer, follow these steps.

1. Access the website you wish to save into your Favorites.
2. Select the Favorites pull-down menu or press the Favorites button.
3. Choose Add to Favorites.

Figure 5.1: Favorites in Microsoft Internet Explorer

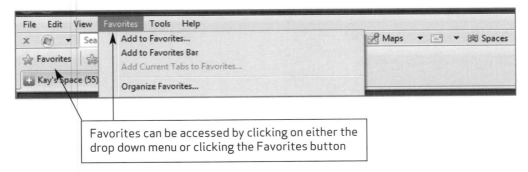

Favorites can be accessed by clicking on either the drop down menu or clicking the Favorites button

4. A dialog box will appear asking you to choose which Favorites folder to add the URL to (or to create a new folder).
5. Select the appropriate folder (or create a new folder) and press OK.
6. The URL will then be added to your Favorites.

Returning to a previously bookmarked website is a simple matter of selecting Favorites (or Bookmarks) and clicking the link to the site you want to visit.

Activity 5.1   *Research*

This activity will enable you to save NHS Evidence as a Favorite by following the steps below.

1. Use Google search to access the NHS Evidence website (**www.evidence.nhs.uk**).

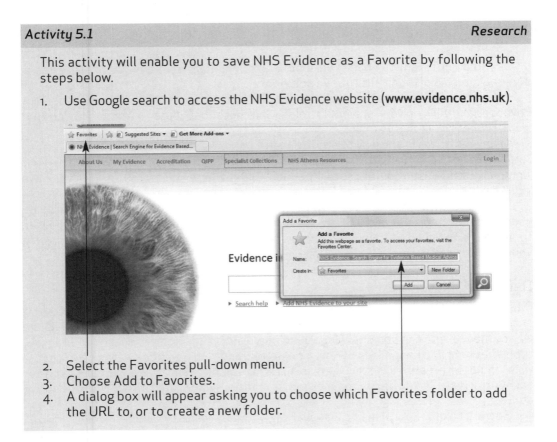

2. Select the Favorites pull-down menu.
3. Choose Add to Favorites.
4. A dialog box will appear asking you to choose which Favorites folder to add the URL to, or to create a new folder.

Activity 5.1 continued

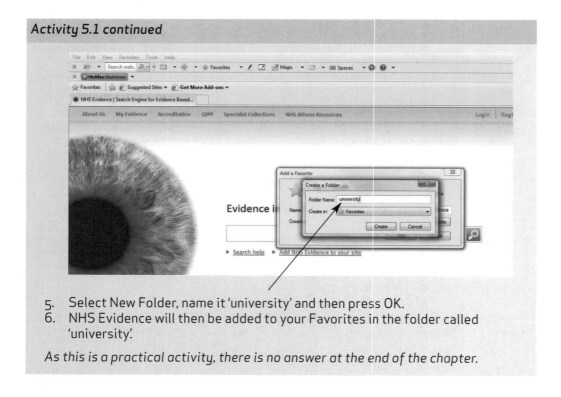

5. Select New Folder, name it 'university' and then press OK.
6. NHS Evidence will then be added to your Favorites in the folder called 'university'.

As this is a practical activity, there is no answer at the end of the chapter.

If you do not want to share your bookmarks and just want a place to store them, personal portals offer an alternative solution.

Now that you have successfully saved NHS Evidence as a Favorite, access your Favorites and click on your 'university' folder and check that your link works. If it does not work, repeat the activity above.

Using Favorites is one way of storing useful websites and you can create a number of folders to make retrieval of information easier. For example, in addition to your 'university' folder, you could create a 'holiday' folder where you store the sites you have visited when planning a holiday.

The one drawback with saving websites in Favorites is that they will be stored on your personal computer and you cannot access them if you log in on another computer, for example, at university. However, there are other systems available that make storing your favourite websites more widely accessible.

Delicious™

Delicious is a free social bookmarking service available at **http://delicious.com**. It enables you to *save all your bookmarks online, share them with other people, and see what other people are bookmarking* (Delicious, 2010). It also offers search and tagging tools that help you keep track of your bookmarks and find new bookmarks from people with similar interests. However, there is no requirement to share and you can keep your account private if you wish. For more information, visit the site itself at the above address.

Social bookmarking also has disadvantages that have been summarised in Table 5.1.

Table 5.1: Advantages and disadvantages of using Delicious

Advantages	Disadvantages
• It allows you to access your bookmarks from any computer that has internet access as the information is stored on the Delicious website. This means you can access your bookmarks and save new ones wherever you can access the internet.	• You need to register for a Yahoo account in order to use the service.
• You can share your bookmarks with fellow students. This may be particularly useful when you are working collaboratively on a project.	• Spammers have started bookmarking the same web page multiple times. This may result in searches delivering unsolicited, often commercial, websites rather than quality ones.
• Delicious can help you find other people who have interesting bookmarks and add their links to your own collection.	
• The service is free.	

Personal portals

A personal portal is a space on the internet that provides a pathway to other content, including bookmarks and many other useful facilities designed around your personal requirements. Personal portals offer an easy way to access and manage online information and communications.

This section will focus on the use of one personal portal called Netvibes™, although others are available such as Pageflakes™, My Yahoo!™, Alot.com™, iGoogle™ and Microsoft Live™.

Netvibes is a free website that lets you personalise your web experience and bring all your online information together in one place. This can include your email accounts, university homepage and virtual learning environment (VLE), as well as online *newspapers, blogs, weather, email, search, videos, photos, social networks, podcasts, widgets, games and funny applications* (Netvibes, 2010). It also provides RSS (Really Simple Syndication – see pages 82–3) facilities.

In order to use Netvibes you need to register an account on the website, but before you consider this visit the Netvibes Overview at **http://tour.netvibes.com/overview.php**. It will give you more information about Netvibes and the range of facilities available as outlined in Figure 5.2.

Figure 5.2: Facilities on Netvibes

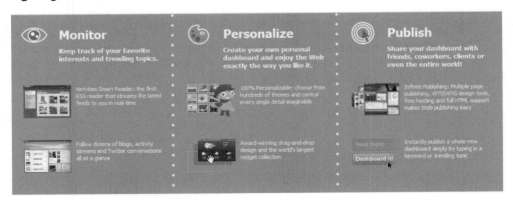

For the purpose of this discussion, access Netvibes at **www.netvibes.com/private page/1#General**. This site provides an example of what a Netvibes page might look like. You can add new tabs to create sections to your Netvibes. You can also change the name of the General tab by double-clicking the tab and overtyping General with the new name.

So that you can see what Netvibes has to offer, I have provided a screenshot of part of my own Netvibes (Figure 5.3). I currently have four sections or tabs in my Netvibes: University, RSS feeds, Personal, and Holidays & travel.

Netvibes is currently open on my University tab, which on my personal PC is set as my home page. On this page I have used the bookmark facility to make links directly to areas I frequently visit, such as my email and library accounts. This page is also home to some general information, such as the local weather, newspapers and BBC Health News.

Figure 5.3: My Netvibes

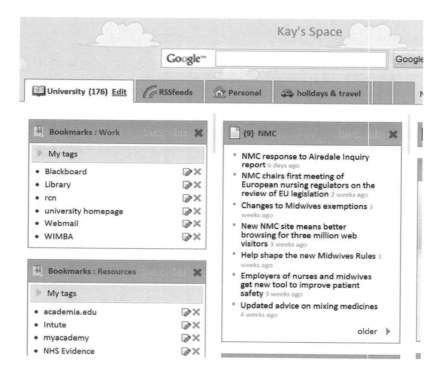

I have found having a personal portal very useful as, when I log on to my Netvibes, I can access work and personal information from one site. Registration is free.

On the left-hand side of my Netvibes (Figure 5.3) you will notice there are two bookmarks: one called Work and the other Resources. If you decide to open a Netvibes account you can place all the most useful bookmarks you have collected and locate them in a similar bookmark in your own Netvibes.

To create bookmarks you need to download a 'bookmark widget' by clicking on the button located in the top left-hand corner of the Netvibes page. This allows access to a drop-down menu (Figure 5.4), from which the Essential widget option can be selected. Then click on Bookmarks.

Once this procedure is completed, the bookmark widget will be added to the top left-hand side of your Netvibes page. You can add a bookmark as often as you like, so you can have different bookmarks for different topics. To use bookmarks in this way you

Figure 5.4: Essential widgets

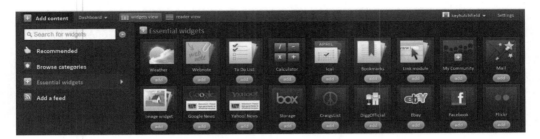

have to use a tag (key word), which tells the widget which bookmark to attach the link to.

Adding your bookmarks is straightforward. Figure 5.5 shows the NHS Evidence bookmark from my Netvibes. I have given the link the title NHS Evidence. The tag is Resources and makes the bookmark appear in my bookmark box that has the tag Resources. If I labelled the tag Holiday, it would add the link to my Holiday bookmarks instead of Resources.

Figure 5.5: Adding a bookmark

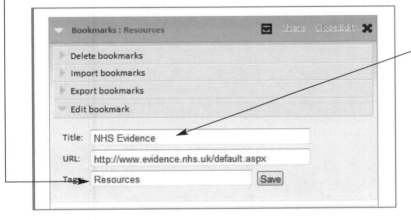

Bookmarks are one way to store and provide quick and easy access to useful or frequently used websites. However, you can also access information by signing up for email alerts.

Email alerts

Some organisations offer the option of regular updates through email alerts. These include alerts from electronic journals and databases, which are a great way to keep up to date with new research in your field, as the database will rerun your search terms on a regular basis without you having to log on to the database. Alerts are particularly useful for anyone working on an extended piece of work, such as a research proposal, literature review or dissertation. Zetoc is just one example.

Zetoc

Zetoc provides access to the British Library's Electronic Table of Contents of around 20,000 current journals and around 16,000 conference proceedings published per year. The database covers 1993 to date, and is updated on a daily basis. It includes an email alerting service, to enable you to keep up-to-date with relevant new articles and papers.

(Zetoc, 2010)

Zetoc is a free service available to universities and the NHS in England, Scotland and Northern Ireland. You can decide how you set up the Zetoc alert to ensure that you maximise the use of the system. You can opt to request to be sent the table of contents from particular journals and/or articles that match particular authors or keywords. Zetoc email alerts can appear as quickly as 72 hours after new material is made available by the publisher. For more information about Zetoc, access their *Frequently Asked Questions* (FAQs) at **http://zetoc.mimas.ac.uk/faq.html**.

The one drawback of using email alerts is that they can block up your email. However, there is a solution: RSS feeds and an aggregator.

RSS feeds

RSS (Really Simple Syndication) is a format for distributing news and other web-based content. Information on an RSS feed is visible as it is updated in the form of headings. Clicking on the headings will lead you to more detailed information on the topic.

The orange and white symbol on the left is used to indicate websites where that page can 'feed' to an aggregator such as Google Reader, or personal portals such as Netvibes, Pageflakes, My Yahoo!, Alot.com, iGoogle and Microsoft Live.

Activity 5.2	Research

This exercise is for those students who are not quite sure what an RSS feed looks like.

1. From your internet browser access the BBC News at **http://news.bbc.co.uk/**.
2. Note the **LATEST** button under the main BBC banner at the top of the page. This section offers information on the very latest news and is continuously updated. Make a note of the key news topics.
3. Click on a heading that interests you and see the additional information available.
4. Print off the front page of the site.
5. Log out.
6. Access the site again in 24 hours.
7. Compare your printout of the front page with the current page and see how much has changed.

As this activity depends on constantly changing information, there is no outline answer at the end of the chapter.

Having visited the BBC website, you can see how convenient a newsfeed can be; it is free, easy to access and current. Like email alerts, RSS feeds bring information to you rather than you having to go and find it.

Recently, the NMC has introduced an RSS feed to their new website. If you return to Figure 5.3 you can see that I have subscribed to this feed and have added it to my Netvibes, so that I have easy access to all the latest news from the NMC every time I log on to the Netvibes.

To use the RSS feed facility you need two things: a home for your information (an aggregator) and sites with an RSS feed facility.

If you have registered for a Netvibes account, RSS feeds can be added by performing the following steps.

1. Click on the 'Add content' button (Figure 5.4).
2. Select the 'Add a feed button' (Figure 5.4).
3. Enter the feed address in the textbox.
4. Press 'Add feed' and the RSS feed will appear on your Netvibes.

Google Reader™

If you do not want to sign up for a personal portal, Google Reader™ feed reader will enable you to create a website where your RSS feeds can be displayed. Google Reader is free and can be accessed at **www.google.com/reader**. This site provides a tour on the front page that explains how Google Reader works and the facilities it provides (Figure 5.6).

As an outcome of your searches, alerts and RSS feeds, you will accumulate an increasing number of references. To keep track of these can be a challenge, but there are ways in which technology can help.

RefWorks

RefWorks™ is an application that helps you manage references by enabling you to create your own bibliographic database of the literature you have found. It is, however, a commercial website for which a subscription is required. If your university holds a subscription, you will be able to access it free of charge.

In addition to providing a storage space where you can manage your references, RefWorks has the facility to generate reference lists and bibliographies. You can also

Figure 5.6: Google Reader

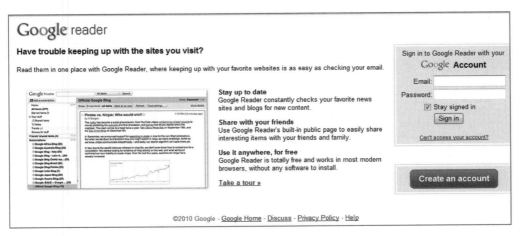

set up RSS feeds from journals so that you can easily import references that are of interest to you.

This is quite a complex tool and attending an introductory workshop is advisable. You will need to practise using it in order to maximise its facilities.

This chapter has provided you with information on how technologies can be used to help you effectively access and manage electronic information. It does not cover all the applications available, but provides a taste of some of the simple and more complex ways in which you can manage the information you need to access for your academic studies and professional practice. It is also designed to assist you in developing good habits that will transfer into your continuing professional development as a registered practitioner.

Check how much you have learnt

Undertake the following short test to see how much you have learnt by completing this chapter. Answers are provided below.

1. Complete the following sentence.
   Favorites or bookmarks can be used to ....
2. Put these instructions on how to create a Favorite in Internet Explorer in the correct order.
   i.   Choose Add to Favorites.
   ii.   Access the website you wish to save into your Favorites.
   iii. Select the appropriate folder (or create a new folder) and press OK.
   iv.   A dialog box will appear asking you to choose which Favorites folder to add the URL to (or to create a new folder).
   v.   Select the Favorites pull-down menu or press the Favorites button.
3. List the four advantages and two disadvantages of using Delicious.

Advantages	Disadvantages
i.	i.
ii.	ii.
iii.	
iv.	

4. Other than bookmarks, name three of the many facilities offered by personal portals such as Netvibes.
   i.
   ii.
   iii.

5. Name one advantage and one disadvantage of email alerts.
   One advantage is ....
   One disadvantage is ....
6. Name the two things you need to use the RSS facility.
   i.
   ii.

Answers

1. Bookmarks (called Favorites in Internet Explorer) allow you to create a record of a web address (URL) and store it on your computer. this enables you to revisit a website without having to remember or write down the address.
2. To create a Favorite in Internet Explorer, the correct steps are as follows.
   i.   Access the website you wish to save into your Favorites.
   ii.   Select the Favorites pull-down menu or press the Favorites button.
   iii. Choose Add to Favorites.
   iv.   A dialog box will appear asking you to choose which Favorites folder to add the URL to (or to create a new folder).
   v.   Select the appropriate folder (or create a new folder) and press OK.
3. The four advantages and two disadvantages of using Delicious are as follows.

Advantages	Disadvantages
i. It allows you to access your bookmarks from any computer that has internet access, as the information is stored on the Delicious website. This means you can access your bookmarks and save new ones whether you are working at home or at university.	i. You need to register for a Yahoo account in order to use the service.
ii. You can share your bookmarks with fellow students. This may be particularly useful when you are working collaboratively on a project.	ii. Spammers have started bookmarking the same web page multiple times. This may result in searches delivering unsolicited, often commercial, websites rather than quality ones.
iii. Delicious can help you find other people who have interesting bookmarks and add their links to your own collection.	
iv. The service is free.	

4. Other than bookmarks, you could have listed any of the following facilities offered by personal portals such as Netvibes.
   Newspapers
   Blogs
   Weather
   News
   Search
   Social networks
   Photos
   Podcasts
   RSS feeds
   And more!
5. Advantages of email alerts you could have included are:
   i.   information comes to you once the alert is set up;
   ii. you can obtain contents pages of your favourite journal;
   iii. they help you keep up to date.
   The main disadvantage is that they may block up your email account.
6. Two things you need to use the RSS facility are:
   i.   a home for your information (an aggregator);
   ii. websites with an RSS feed facility.

Knowledge review

Having completed the chapter, how would you now rate your knowledge of the following topics?

	Good	Adequate	Poor
1. How to store web addresses.			
2. How to sign up for email alerts.			
3. How personal portals can provide easy access to information.			

Where you're not confident in your knowledge of a topic, what will you do next?

Useful websites

www.evidence.nhs.uk NHS Evidence – take the tour and then create your own space.
www.youtube.com/watch?v=VSPZ2Uu_X3Y An easy-to-understand short video about Google Reader.
http://delicious.com
http://alot.com Alot personal portal
http://delicious.com Delicious free social bookmarking service
www.google.com/ig iGoogle personal portal
www.google.com/reader Online aggregator of RSS and other feeds
www.live.com Microsoft Live personal portal
http://my.yahoo.com My Yahoo! personal portal
www.netvibes.com Netvibes personal portal
www.pageflakes.com Pageflakes personal portal
www.refworks.com Online tool for managing references and RSS journal feeds
http://zetoc.mimas.ac.uk Zetoc journal article email alert service and database

Chapter 6

Health informatics and continuing professional development

Draft NMC Standards for Pre-registration Nursing Education

This chapter will address the following draft competencies:

Domain: Communication and interpersonal skills

2. All nurses must use a range of communication skills and technologies and to support person-centred care and enhance the quality and safety of healthcare. They must make sure that people receive all the information they need about their care in a language and manner that is right for them, and that allows them to make informed choices and consent to treatment.

Domain: Nursing practice and decision making

8. All nurses must make person-centred, evidence-based judgements and decisions, in partnership with others involved in the care process, to ensure that quality care is delivered.

Domain: Leadership, management and team working

10. All nurses must draw on a range of resources to evaluate and audit care, and then use this information to contribute to improving people's experience and outcomes of care and the shaping of future services.

Draft Essential Skills Clusters

This chapter will address the following draft ESCs:

Cluster: Organisational aspects of care

10. People can trust the newly registered graduate nurse to deliver nursing interventions and evaluate their effectiveness against the agreed assessment and care plan.

By the second progression point:

iv. Actively seeks to extend knowledge and skills using a variety of methods in order to enhance care delivery.

Chapter aims

After reading this chapter, you will be able to:

- outline the nature of health informatics and how it is used to enhance care;
- identify how health informatics influences the continuing professional development needs of student and registered nurses.

Introduction

In the first chapter of this book the need to develop IT skills was linked to the key skills identified in the Dearing Report as essential transferable skills for effective learning. This chapter focuses on illustrating why these key transferable skills are increasingly needed by professionals working in healthcare to access the evidence needed to underpin professional practice. It will introduce you to the concept of health informatics and why this is becoming an increasingly important area of development for all staff working within the NHS.

Introduction to health informatics

All NHS staff should have basic IT skills and an understanding of relevant legislation to support their involvement in the increasing use of technology within the health service. Health informatics involves far more than just computer skills. NHS Careers (2010) describes health informatics as *an emerging discipline within healthcare* and defines it as:

> The knowledge, skills and tools which enable information to be collected, managed, used and shared to support the delivery of healthcare and to promote health.

However, the focus for this book is on finding, accessing and evaluating information rather than issues of copyright, privacy and data protection.

This book has focused on one aspect of health informatics – the use of technology to facilitate the access, storage and retrieval of information, in order to keep up to date in a health environment that has an expectation that clinical decisions will be based on the most recent evidence and guidelines. However, health informatics is a wider concept that recognises the need of health services to be responsive, easily accessible and resource efficient.

Health informatics is concerned with using technology to improve the speed and efficiency of processing and communicating information related to patients' care, such as requesting and accessing laboratory tests, prescriptions and X-rays. It is concerned with developing systems to manage routine tasks, such as ordering supplies, booking appointments and communication. In many ways, health informatics should be a means of freeing up more time for health professionals to deliver direct care that is underpinned by the most recent evidence.

CASE STUDY: Choose and book

Below are some examples of patient perspectives on the new system for managing outpatient appointments called 'Choose and Book'; the examples are taken from the NHS Connecting for Health website.

- 'The Choose and Book system is a radical improvement on the old paper system,' says Mike. 'As a busy professional, I need to manage my time carefully. Choose and Book made it so much easier to book an appointment and made sure that I got one that fitted in well with my busy schedule.'
- 'It has really felt like a service that can accommodate my needs as an individual and not something where I have to fall in line.'
- 'I've been absolutely delighted with it [Choose and Book]. I think Choose and Book is much better than the old paper system. It's lovely knowing that you're going to get to see someone and exactly when you're going to see them.'

These examples suggest that Choose and Book provides a more person-focused service that offers the patient more choice. It may also result in a reduction in the numbers of patients who fail to attend their appointments as patients can choose appointment times most convenient for them.

However, using technology does not just benefit the patient, as you can see from the following Case Study, from Sarah, a junior sister on an acute ward within a general district hospital.

CASE STUDY: Patient Centre

'Patient Centre is a computer program that centralises everything that a patient may need during their treatment at the hospital. It enables you to search for patients to see their past admission history; when patients are admitted as inpatients or ward attendees, it enables you to order haematology, biochemistry, microbiology or pathology tests; and you can order specialist therapies, e.g. physiotherapy or occupational therapy. You can organise outpatient appointments, and transfers to and from the hospital or to other hospitals. You can track, request or find notes and access waiting lists from there too. This is a useful system as everything is now in one place with one password, rather than having to access several different systems.

We also have a new system called Telepathology Link, which displays all the results of haematology, biochemistry, microbiology or pathology. It is quick and easy to use and means you no longer have to wait for the labs to phone you with the results. Now they are often on the system in 1–2 hours.'

As you can see from Sarah's comments, the use of technology makes the access to information much quicker. Nurses no longer need to telephone laboratories for results, and technicians can spend their time processing test results rather than answering telephone enquiries or telephoning through results.

A brief history of the development of health informatics in the UK

In 1998, the Department of Health (DH) published *Information for Health*, which committed the NHS to developing 24-hour access to electronic patient records and making information about the best clinical practice available to all who worked within the NHS.

In 2002, the Wanless Report made recommendations for the financing, standards and management of IT implementation in the NHS. This report and the subsequent publication of *Delivering 21st Century IT Support for the NHS* (DH, 2002) laid the foundations for the National Programme for IT, with the aim of developing an integrated IT infrastructure and system for all NHS organisations in England. In April 2005, Connecting for Health was established, which combined responsibility for the delivery of the National Programme with the IT-related functions of the NHS Information Authority under one organisation. This ensured a more coordinated approach that is more responsive to the needs of patients and practitioners, and focused on improving the speed and efficiency of the service provided.

NHS Connecting for Health

NHS Connecting for Health provides computer-assisted systems and services designed to improve the way NHS patient information is stored and accessed (NHS Connecting for Health, 2010). There are many aspects to the work of NHS Connecting for Health and Table 6.1 provides a brief summary of the main activities.

Comprehensive details of all the activities of NHS Connecting for Health can be found under the Systems and Services section of the Connecting for Health website at **www.connectingforhealth.nhs.uk/systemsandservices**. The site offers examples of patient experiences of some of these systems.

PACS offers a more efficient system for managing and storing scans and X-rays. In addition to reducing the need for physical storage space, it also reduces the likelihood of scans and X-rays being lost as they are stored electronically. The following Case Study is a summary of one patient's experience of PACS and is an extract from an example on the NHS Connecting for Health website. It illustrates how PACS can enhance care and increase patient satisfaction. The patient concerned was a doctor who had broken his leg in a skiing accident.

CASE STUDY: PACS

What also struck me was the speed with which the X-ray images were produced and shared, and the confidence the clinicians demonstrated in using the system. There were no delays, no carrying around packets of films. The efficiency was impressive and I even have a digital copy of my images as a souvenir!

Availability of the same images at my local clinic also enabled my physiotherapist to provide the best advice immediately, reducing my recovery time.

When I think about how it took just a few minutes for my son to upload a digital photo on to the web, it brought home to me that PACS really is appropriate for the digital age. It's helping us to take healthcare into the twenty-first century and, as a clinician, I am excited about using this and other technological developments to improve care and involve patients more.'

Table 6.1: Main services and systems provided through NHS Connecting for Health (2010)

Service or system	Description
NHS Care Record Service	This service is aimed at providing a Summary Care record and a Detailed Care record for every consenting patient using the NHS. It aims to provide a secure service that electronically links patient information from different parts of the NHS.
PACS (Picture Archiving and Communication System)	PACS provides a digital storage system for images such as X-rays and scans that enables them to be stored electronically and viewed on screens. This system allows the immediate sharing of images with specialist services without the need for the physical transfer of films or patients.
EPS (Electronic Prescription Service)	The EPS will enable prescribers (such as GPs and practice nurses) to send prescriptions electronically to a pharmacy of the patient's choice. This will make the prescribing and dispensing process safer and more convenient for patients and staff.
AIDC (Automatic Identification and Data Capture)	This system uses bar codes and radio frequency technology to increase patient safety in the NHS. The main areas relate to patient identification through the use of bar codes, prevention of prescription and drug administration errors, and the tracking and tracing of instruments, equipment and patient records.
NHS Patient Pathways	NHS Patient Pathways capacity management system is designed for use in any emergency or urgent care telephone assessment setting, such as the ambulance service, NHS Direct and GP out-of-hours services. It is a tool for triaging telephone calls from the public, using a structured symptom-based flow chart and based on the symptoms people report when they call in.
Clinical Dashboard	A Clinical Dashboard is a display tool that provides clinicians with relevant and timely information to inform daily decisions that improve the quality of patient care. The displays give clinicians easy access to a wealth of data, chosen by them to meet their local requirements, in a highly visible and usable format.

Developing relevant IT skills

Given these developments, it is obviously important that you continue to develop your IT skills to progress your career in future healthcare. If you have grown up in the digital age, transferring and developing your IT skills in healthcare is unlikely to be problematic. However, you will still need to ensure you understand the principles of data protection, privacy and copyright. If you are a mature student or simply not 'computer-minded', you may initially find it difficult to motivate yourself to develop the necessary IT skills you need for your practice. Perhaps this Case Study may help you to feel motivated.

CASE STUDY: Developing IT skills

Ruby was a 43-year-old woman who had been qualified as a nurse for 24 years. She worked in a busy ophthalmic department and had decided she wanted to undertake her mentorship programme. However, her manager insisted that Ruby attend an academic development module before embarking on her mentorship programme, as she had not participated in any formal study since qualifying.

Initially, Ruby was very anxious about the module and was particularly resistant to the idea of developing her IT skills. As the module progressed, Ruby began to realise that using technology could help her access a wider range of information to support her practice.

In her final essay Ruby stated that not only had her IT skills improved, but she was actively seeking further development as she realised that by developing these skills she could enhance her practice. She was now able to access electronic patient records and laboratory results, and make appointments and referrals electronically, rather than having to ask her colleagues to do these tasks for her. This had resulted in an increase in Ruby's level of confidence at work and she felt motivated to continue to develop her practice.

NHS Connecting for Health also offers information about free IT training for NHS staff. Currently part of this provision is delivered in collaboration with Microsoft through NHS Microsoft IT Academies, which are located in each strategic health authority (SHA) in England.

In addition, some basic IT programmes are available through the Essential IT Skills (EITS) Programme. The EITS Programme addresses two areas of learning.

- NHS ELITE (eLearning IT Essentials): trains staff on basic keyboard and mouse skills as well as file management, web and email skills.
- NHS Health (eLearning for Health Information Systems): gives staff the training they need to ensure that they comply with information governance, data protection and patient confidentiality requirements.

Activity 6.1 *Reflection*

- How confident are you that you have the necessary basic IT skills to work within health and social care? How did you score in Activity 1.5 in Chapter 1 (page 15)?
- How confident are you in using Microsoft Office programmes such as:
  - word processing (Word);
  - databases (Excel and Access);
  - presentation programmes (PowerPoint and Publisher)?
- What action have you planned to improve these skills?
- Review the personal development plan (PDP) you created in Chapter 1 (see pages 16–18). Have you included improving your skills in using these programmes in your plan?
- Do you need to seek any further help from your university study support department in the light of this reflection?
- Amend your PDP so that it takes into consideration your reflections.

As this activity is based on your own skills development, there is no outline answer at the end of the chapter.

National Occupational Standards

During your nursing programme the standards and competencies you need to develop are determined by the NMC and the Quality Assurance Agency (QAA). Each of these organisations monitors universities to ensure that the programmes they offer will enable nursing students to meet their standards and competencies.

Once you have qualified and are registered as a practitioner in your field of practice, the NMC will continue to guide and monitor your performance through *The Code*, guidelines, consultations, circulars and the re-registration and Fitness for Practice processes.

Both the NMC and Department of Health have a clear focus on the delivery of good-quality care to service users. Once you are employed as a nurse you will be expected to make a commitment to 'lifelong learning' and to comply with the National Occupational Standards (NOS) for your profession. For nurses, these standards are embedded within the Knowledge and Skills Framework.

The Knowledge and Skills Framework

The Knowledge and Skills Framework (KSF) is a competency-based framework designed to promote quality care provision through personal development, appraisal and career progression (RCN, 2005). It defines and describes the knowledge and skills that NHS staff need for a particular post and is intended to support staff so that they can be effective in their jobs. In addition to supporting learning, the KSF is linked to pay progression.

The KSF was implemented in 2004, but there is limited reference made to health informatics skills other than in the context of nurses in specialist research roles or management. However, more recent government policy, such as *A High Quality Workforce: NHS next stage review* (DH, 2008), provides a stronger focus on linking clinical practice, academic development and the use of the best available evidence to enhance practice.

A High Quality Workforce

Some statements from *A High Quality Workforce* (DH, 2008) have been presented in Table 6.2 to illustrate that the nurse of the future will need to have a reasonable level of information-handling skills and IT competence to access and utilise IT systems, such as those being developed in NHS Connecting for Health.

Regardless of the framework, proficiency with IT is an essential transferable skill that supports the professional practice of nurses in the twenty-first century. A Case Study of my own experience as a patient may illustrate this.

CASE STUDY: *IT supporting practice*

In 2007, I developed a painful skin condition on my hands. My GP referred me to the local NHS dermatologist and I was invited to attend a nurse-led assessment clinic three weeks later. During the assessment the nurse took a series of digital photographs of the affected areas of skin on my hands.

She explained that the dermatologist would review the assessment information the nurse had gathered and look at the photographs. The dermatologist would decide on one of two courses of action. Either he would contact my GP and recommend a course of treatment or he would ask me to attend his clinic for further examination.

This seemed a very sensible way of making use of the skills of the nurse and of technology to allow the dermatologist to focus on the more serious and challenging cases.

Table 6.2: Extracts from *A High Quality Workforce*: NHS next stage review

Statement	IT skills required
23. Promoting life-long learning: Staff in all roles and settings need opportunities to continuously update the skills and techniques that are relevant to delivering high-quality care through, for example, work-based learning, distance and e-learning, and further education.	In order to engage in distance and e-learning, practitioners will need to be able to use the internet, virtual learning environments and email.
52. Support systems: IT systems that deliver necessary information in timely fashion.	Practitioners will need to be confident in the use of some transferable and basic IT skills in order to engage with information systems, such as those outlined in NHS Connecting for Health.
54. Stronger clinical academic careers that combine research and education with clinical careers to improve the translation of research into clinical practice. We will continue the work we have begun to implement the recommendations of the UK Clinical Research Collaboration so that we integrate clinical and academic nursing careers. We will undertake further work focusing on nurse educators.	Practitioners who wish to combine research and education will need advanced IT skills that will enable them to access evidence and utilise statistical analysis tools to enhance data analysis. Use of NHS intranet and electronic communication can also assist in the engagement in and dissemination of evidence to others.

Source: Department of Health (2008, pp13, 19–20).

Preceptorship

A High Quality Workforce (DH, 2008) also acknowledges the fact that the end of any pre-registration nursing programme is not the end of learning but the beginning of another phase of lifelong learning.

A number of studies have been undertaken that suggest that the transition from student to registered nurse is not straightforward (Ross and Clifford, 2002; Clark and Holmes, 2007; Mooney, 2007) and that appropriate support can improve the experience of transition and retention of newly qualified staff (Mooney, 2007). This evidence is reflected in the commitment to improve the provision of a period of preceptorship for newly qualified nurses.

> *54. Threefold increase in investment in foundation periods. A foundation period of preceptorship for nurses at the start of their careers will help them begin the journey from novice to expert. This will enable them to apply knowledge, skills and competences acquired as students, into their area of practice, laying a solid foundation for life-long learning. As a first step, we will increase threefold the amount currently invested to provide newly qualified staff with protected time and other support as they move into practice for the first time.*
>
> (DH, 2008, p19)

This commitment to provide support for the transition from student to independent practitioner is welcomed. Protected time for clinical supervision and/or reflection with a preceptor would seem to be an important feature if preceptorship is to be effective. Perhaps technology will be part of the solution through the development of blogs and Twitter.

Lifelong learning and continuing professional development

The NMC also has an expectation that nurses will continue to learn and develop their knowledge and skills throughout their working lives.

The Code (NMC, 2008a), under the heading 'Keep your skills and knowledge up to date' states that, as a nurse, you must:

- have the knowledge and skills for safe and effective practice when working without direct supervision;
- recognise and work within the limits of your competence;
- keep your knowledge and skills up to date throughout your working life;
- take part in appropriate learning and practice activities that maintain and develop your competence and performance.

Once you are qualified you will no longer have the university to set targets for you, and you will have to take full responsibility for your learning and keeping up to date with new evidence and changes in practice. It is here that well-established information skills will be beneficial, especially if you are also working full-time, when fitting in time for activities that will enable you to keep up to date may be a challenge.

If you develop good study habits and have established effective information skills during your time at university, you will find it easier to find the time to continue professional development activities once you are qualified. As a registered nurse, you will need well-developed information skills to access the evidence that will form the basis of your practice and to make use of the IT systems in your place of work.

Below are some ideas of how you can expand the good study and information skills habits you developed in university into your practice as a qualified nurse.

1. Making good use of your time in and out of work.
    - Always make a plan *before* you begin a search for information.
    - Create a list of reliable sources of evidence that provide the best evidence for your particular field of practice (e.g. bibliographic databases, information gateways or e-journals), so that finding information becomes a reasonably quick activity.
    - Plan reading time into each week so that you make use of small pockets of time (typically 40–60 minutes) that might otherwise be wasted (e.g. on bus or train journeys, waiting to pick up children/friends/family, or over a cup of tea in the morning or evening.
    - Subscribe to a relevant professional journal and join a local journal club if one exists in your locality.
    - Attend in-house training, workshops and seminars offered within your practice area.
    - Where available in your workplace, make use of clinical supervision or reflection with colleagues to learn from clinical experiences.

2. Use technology to access, store and retrieve information effectively.
   - Store useful web links as bookmarks in Favorites or social bookmarking services such a Delicious.
   - Make use of email alerts to bring the latest information to you.
   - Set up your own personal portal so that you can use selected RSS feeds to bring information relating to your field of practice directly to you.

Easy access to current evidence will enable you to develop and extend your knowledge base, improve your ability to develop your nursing career, and deliver care that is based on the best available evidence. This is not only an expectation of the NMC but of the public.

The subject of evidenced-based practice in nursing is explored further in another book in this series.

C H A P T E R S U M M A R Y

This chapter has considered the nature of health informatics and how it has developed through the work of NHS Connecting for Health. It has demonstrated how the information skills outlined in this book are necessary for effective functioning within any healthcare workforce, and how study habits developed in university can form a sound basis for lifelong learning within professional practice.

Check how much you have learnt

Undertake the following short test to see how much you have learnt by completing this chapter. Answers are provided below.

1. Complete the following statement.
   Health informatics is defined as the ...., ... and .... that enable information to be ...., ..., ... and .... to support the delivery of healthcare and to promote health.
2. List three of the main services and systems provided by NHS Connecting for Health.
   i.
   ii.
   iii.
3. Which of the following statements is correct?
   i.   NHS Elite offers an introduction to Microsoft Office.
   ii. NHS Health provides training on data protection.
   iii. Every SHA in England has a Microsoft IT Academy.
4. List four ways in which good information skills can help you make good use of the time you have to study.
   i.
   ii.
   iii.
   iv.
5. Name three ways in which technology can be used to improve the access, storage and retrieval of information.
   i.
   ii.
   iii.

Answers

1. Health informatics is defined as the *knowledge, skills* and *tools* that enable information to be *collected, managed, used* and *shared* to support the delivery of healthcare and to promote health.
2. Your list of the main services and systems provided by NHS Connecting for Health should have included three of the following.
   NHS Care Record Service
   PACS (Picture Archiving and Communication System)
   EPS (Electronic Prescription Service)
   AIDC (Automatic Identification and Data Capture)
   NHS Patient Pathways
   Clinical Dashboard
3. The following statements are correct.
   ii. NHS Health provides training on data protection.
   iii. Every SHA in England has a Microsoft IT Academy.
4. Effective information skills can help you make good use of the time you have to study by:
   i.   ensuring effective use of the time available by:
        - effective planning of searches;
        - knowing where to look for information;
   ii. giving you the ability to use a range of information sources provided by your university and NHS;
   iii. providing good systems for effective storage and easy retrieval of information
   iv. making use of technology (e.g. RSS feeds and email alerts) to bring information to you.
5. Technology can improve the access, storage or retrieval of information by:
   i.   allowing you to store web sources using facilities such as Favorites or Delicious;
   ii. the use of RefWorks to store references;
   iii. allowing you to set up a personal portal such as Netvibes to bring together all the information you need to access in one place.

Knowledge review

Having completed the chapter, how would you now rate your knowledge of the following topics?

		Good	Adequate	Poor
1.	The definition and history of health informatics.			
2.	NHS Connecting for Health services and systems.			
3.	National Occupational Standards for nursing.			
4.	Preceptorship, lifelong learning and CPD.			

Where you're not confident in your knowledge of a topic, what will you do next?

Further reading

Hannah, K, Ball, M and Edwards, M (eds) *Introduction to Nursing Informatics*. London: Springer.

Useful websites

www.connectingforhealth.nhs.uk/systemsandservices NHS Connecting for Health information about the IT training available to support health professionals. On this page, enter 'EITS' into the search box for more on Essential IT Skills.

www.nmc-uk.org On the NMC home page, type 'preceptorship' into the search box to access the Preceptorship Guidelines (Circular 21/2006).

References

Clark, T and Holmes, S (2007) Fit for practice? An exploration of the development of newly qualified nurses using focus groups. *International Journal of Nursing Studies* 44(7): 1210–20.

Dearing, Ron (1997) *The National Committee of Inquiry into Higher Education.* Available online at https://bei.leeds.ac.uk/Partners/NCIHE/ (accessed 13 June 2010).

Delicious (2010) *Home Page.* Available online at http://delicious.com/ (accessed 13 June 2010).

Department of Health (DH) (1998) *Information for Health.* London: Department of Health, NHS Executive. Available online at http://www.dh.gov.uk/en/Publicationsand statistics/Publications/PublicationsPolicyAndGuidance/DH_4002944.

Department of Health (DH) (2002) *Delivering 21st Century IT Support for the NHS.* London: Department of Health.

Department of Health (DH) (2007) *Managing Attrition Rates for Student Nurses and Midwives.* London: Department of Health. Available online at http://www.dh.gov.uk/en/Publicationsandstatistics/Publications/PublicationsPolicyAndGuidance/DH_073 230 (accessed 13 June 2010).

Department of Health (DH) (2008) *A High Quality Workforce: NHS next stage review.* Available online at www.dh.gov.uk/en/Publicationsandstatistics/Publications/PublicationsPolicyAndGuidance/DH_085840 (accessed 1 June 2010).

Evans, M (2003) *Personal Development Planning: An essential guide.* London: RCN Publishing.

Gibbs, G (1988) *Learning by Doing: A guide to teaching and learning methods.* Oxford: Oxford Brookes University.

Google Scholar (2010) *Help.* Available online at www.google.com/support/scholar/bin/request.py (accessed 31 May 2010).

Haig, K, Sutton, S and Whittingham, J (2006) SBAR: a shared model of improving communication between clinicians. *Journal of Quality and Patient Safety*, 32(3): 167–75.

Jasper, M (2006) *Reflection, Decision-Making and Professional Development.* Oxford: Blackwell.

Laming, Lord (2003) *The Victoria Climbié Inquiry.* London: Crown Publications.

Mindtools (2009) *SWOT Analysis.* Available online at www.mindtools.com/pages/article/newTMC_05.htm (accessed 13 June 2010).

Mooney, M (2007) Facing registration: the expectations and the unexpected. *Nurse Education Today*, 27(8): 840–7.

National Patient Safety Agency (NPSA) (2007) *Recognising and Responding Appropriately to Early Signs of Deterioration in Hospitalised Patients.* Available online at www.npsa.nhs.uk/corporate/news/deterioration-in-hospitalised-patients/ (accessed 13 June 2010).

Netvibes (2010) *Overview*. Available online at http://tour.netvibes.com/overview.php (accessed 12 June 2010).

NHS Careers (2010) *Careers in Health Informatics*. Available online at www.nhs careers.nhs.uk/details/Default.aspx?Id=767 (accessed 13 June 2010).

NHS Connecting for Health (2010) *About Us*. Available online at www.connecting forhealth.nhs.uk/about (accessed 13 June 2010).

NHS Evidence (2010) *Health Information Resources*. Available online at www.library. nhs.uk (accessed 31 May 2010).

Nursing and Midwifery Council (NMC) (2004) *Standards and Proficiencies for Pre-registration Nursing Education*. London: NMC.

Nursing and Midwifery Council (NMC) (2007) *Essential Skills Clusters*. London: NMC.

Nursing and Midwifery Council (NMC) (2008a) *The Code: Standards of conduct, performance and ethics for nurses and midwives*. London: NMC.

Nursing and Midwifery Council (NMC) (2008b) *Your Code of Conduct Applies to your Personal Life*. Available online at www.medicalnewstoday.com/articles/130310.php (accessed 13 June 2010).

Nursing and Midwifery Council (NMC) (2009) *Record Keeping: Guidance for nurses and midwives*. London: NMC. Available online at www.nmc-uk.org/Documents/Guidance/ nmcGuidanceRecordKeepingGuidanceforNursesandMidwives.pdf (accessed 13 June 2010).

Nursing and Midwifery Council (NMC) (2010) *Standards for Pre-registration Nursing Education*. London: NMC.

Office of National Statistics (ONS) (2010) *Home Page*. Available online at www. statistics.gov.uk (accessed 12 May 2010).

Quality and Assurance Agency (QAA) (2001) *Subject Benchmark Statements*. Available online at www.qaa.ac.uk/academicinfrastructure/benchmark/default.asp (accessed 13 June 2010).

Ross, H and Clifford, K (2002) Research as a catalyst for change: the transition from student to Registered Nurse. *Journal of Clinical Nursing*, 11: 545–53.

Royal College of Nursing (RCN) (2005) *NHS Knowledge and Skills Framework Outlines for Nursing Posts*. Available online at www.rcn.org.uk/_data/assets/pdf_file/0007/ 78667/002775.pdf (accessed 1 June 2010).

Rycroft-Malone, J, Seers, K, Titchen, A, Harvey, G, Kitson, A and McCormack, B (2004) An exploration of the factors that influence the implementation of evidence into practice. *Journal of Clinical Nursing*, 13: 913–24.

Truss, L (2003) *Eats, Shoots and Leaves*. London: Profile Books.

University of Sheffield (2010) *Hierarchy of Evidence*. Available online at www.hse. ie/eng/about/Who/Population_Health/Health_Intelligence/Health_Intelligence_Work /Evidence_Based_Health_Care/Hierarchy_of_Evidence/ (accessed 13 June 2010).

Wanless, Derek (2002) *Securing Our Future Health: Taking a long-term view: Final report*. London: HM Treasury. Available online at http://webarchive.nationalarchives.gov.uk (accessed 31 May 2010).

Wikipedia (2010) *Home Page*. Available online at http://en.wikipedia.org/wiki/Main_Page (accessed 31 May 2010).

Wojciechowicz, L (2010) *Internet for Nursing*, free online tutorial, The Virtual Learning Suite (formerly owned by The Intute Consortium). Available online at www.vts.intute.ac.uk/tutorial/nursing (accessed 31 May 2010).

Yorke, M and Longden, B (2008) *The First-year Experience of Higher Education in the UK: Final report*. York: The Higher Education Academy.

Zetoc (2010) *Home Page*. Available online at http://zetoc.mimas.ac.uk/faq.html (accessed 31 May 2010).

Index

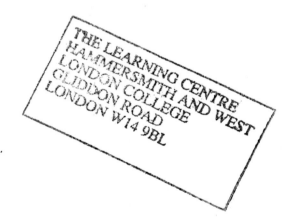